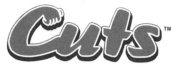

If this book is meant as a "gift of health," please use this page as a dedication.

—JOHN GENNARO

Cuts
FITNESS FOR MEN

The Ultimate 30-Minute Workout

John Gennaro

WITH Myatt Murphy AND Steven Haase

A PERIGEE BOOK

A PERIGEE BOOK
Published by the Penguin Group
Penguin Group (USA) Inc.
375 Hudson Street, New York, New York 10014, USA

Penguin Group (Canada), 90 Eglinton Avenue East, Suite 700, Toronto, Ontario M4P 2Y3, Canada (a division of Pearson Penguin Canada Inc.) • Penguin Books Ltd., 80 Strand, London WC2R 0RL, England • Penguin Group Ireland, 25 St. Stephen's Green, Dublin 2, Ireland (a division of Penguin Books Ltd.) • Penguin Group (Australia), 250 Camberwell Road, Camberwell, Victoria 3124, Australia (a division of Pearson Australia Group Pty. Ltd.) • Penguin Books India Pvt. Ltd., 11 Community Centre, Panchsheel Park, New Dehli—110 017, India • Penguin Group (NZ), 67 Apollo Drive, Rosedale, North Shore 0745, Auckland, New Zealand (a division of Pearson New Zealand Ltd.) • Penguin Books (South Africa) (Pty.) Ltd., 24 Sturdee Avenue, Rosebank, Johannesburg 2196, South Africa

Penguin Books Ltd., Registered Offices: 80 Strand, London WC2R 0RL, England

While the author has made every effort to provide accurate telephone numbers and Internet addresses at the time of publication, neither the publisher nor the author assumes any responsibility for errors, or for changes that occur after publication. Further, the publisher does not have any control over and does not assume any responsibility for author or third-party websites or their content.

CUTS FITNESS FOR MEN

First edition: May 2007

Perigee trade paperback ISBN: 978-0-399-53341-9

An application to register this book for cataloging has been submitted to the Library of Congress.

PRINTED IN THE UNITED STATES OF AMERICA

10 9 8 7 6 5 4 3 2 1

PUBLISHER'S NOTE: Neither the publisher nor the author is engaged in rendering professional advice or services to the individual reader. The ideas, procedures, and suggestions contained in this book are not intended as a substitute for consulting with your physician. All matters regarding your health require medical supervision. Neither the author nor the publisher shall be liable or responsible for any loss or damage allegedly arising from any information or suggestion in this book.

Most Perigee books are available at special quantity discounts for bulk purchases for sales promotions, premiums, fund-raising, or educational use. Special books, or book excerpts, can also be created to fit specific needs. For details, write: Special Markets, Penguin Group (USA) Inc., 375 Hudson Street, New York, New York 10014.

CONTENTS

FOREWORD

As a heart surgeon, I spend much of my career treating the major life-threatening complication of being out of shape: coronary artery disease. Many of my patients have accumulated fat around their waists that directly causes high blood pressure, out-of-control cholesterol, and dangerous levels of blood sugar.

That's the problem. The cure?

It's something that's completely under your control, yet it remains as elusive as a behind-the-fridge roach. It's exercise. We need to exercise. One reason is because your capacity to exercise is a great predictor of how young (and long) you will live. But we also need to do it in order to lose weight. The trick, however, is that we need to do more than just run, cycle, or play hoops to work and strengthen our hearts. We need to move some weight to work and strengthen our muscles.

Here's a fact: muscle burns fifty times more calories than fat. So to lose that dangerous belly fat around your waist, you need to build muscle in other parts of your body. So why isn't everyone squatting, pressing, and lifting? For one, folks give more excuses than a homework-forgetting teenager. No time, no money, no energy, no equipment, no clean spandex. So how do we combat that mind-set? With programs that are efficient and also stimulate a sense of community and obligation, so that participants sense peer pressure to continue to show up (even on days when they'd rather do crunches with their mouths than with their abdominals). We need a way to ensure that you don't skip even once. Because once turns to twice and twice turns to developing TV-induced couch sores. When you skip even one workout, you say that you'll start next month. But, as we all well know, procrastination works about as well as a one-legged bar stool.

John Gennaro has found the way to break this yo-yo cycle of inactivity by designing an insightful solution. Cuts Fitness For Men is a men's-only fitness franchise—it provides men who are out of shape or just getting into shape with a quick and effective workout in a comfortable environment. It features a 30-minute circuit-training-workout standard that appeals to the masses of men who are not currently involved in regular exercise. In effect, Cuts is helping in the battle against obesity by building the muscle that burns through our fat stores. Through Cuts, thousands of men are being introduced to fitness, and in an affordable and supportive atmosphere that men become very passionate about. Cuts is doing for men what Curves and other women's-only fitness franchises have done for millions of women over the last decade.

Now, we have the outline to the Cuts program. John Gennaro wrote the *Cuts Fitness For Men* book to provide a succinct guide to finding fitness and a healthy lifestyle. Readers will identify with John's story of personally making the switch to fitness as an average guy. The Cuts philosophy comes alive as you understand the motivation of its many members. Core topics of the book include strength and cardio training information, including sample workouts. But John also delves into the physiology of health and explains the importance of knowing your target heart rate and the rejuvenating impact of sleep. He also recognizes the need for some men to see their doctor, especially if their butt/waist ratio predicts significant future health issues.

The book is packed with member testimonials from men representing all ages and sizes who have experienced success with the program. I applaud John Gennaro and Cuts Fitness For Men for finally being able to connect with the "Average Joe" who has typically shunned all forms of exercise. After all, when you start moving it, you'll start losing it.

—Mehmet C. Oz, M.D.

About Dr. Mehmet Oz

Mehmet C. Oz, M.D., is the professor and vice chairman of surgery at Columbia University and director of the Cardiovascular Institute and medical director for the Complementary Medicine Program at New York Presbyterian Hospital. Dr. Oz is a widely published author, including the award-winning *Healing from the Heart* and three bestselling books, *YOU: The Owner's Manual*, *YOU: The Smart Patient*, and *YOU: On a Diet*. He has written numerous articles for consumer and medical publications, including regular columns for *Reader's Digest*, *Esquire*, and *O: The Oprah Magazine*. He is also a host on the XM Satellite Radio show *Oprah and Friends*.

ONE

ARE YOU READY TO TURN BACK TIME?

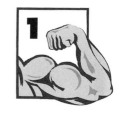

YOU'RE NEVER TOO OLD TO FEEL YOUNG

Men come in all shapes and sizes.

Maybe you're a guy in his thirties, with a little more weight around your middle than you had five years ago. Perhaps you're a guy who some say is well past his prime, but you know you're still young at heart. You just want to look and feel that way again. Or are you a guy that's never known what it's like to be in better shape? You've always wanted to be, but you just didn't know how. Or maybe you're already in the best shape of your life, but looking for a more convenient method to stay that way.

The truth is, it doesn't matter who you are, what your age is or even what your goals are. It doesn't even matter how you first heard of Cuts Fitness For Men and the book you're about to read. As the president and founder of Cuts Fitness—the worldwide chain of fitness facilities that's been showing men how to finally make time for exercise—I've noticed that it's not how someone gets introduced to fitness, it's how they introduce fitness into their own lives.

Get Ready to Change Your Life

Today, I am pleased to say that Cuts Fitness For Men is the fastest growing men's fitness franchise in the world, having garnered worldwide attention from publications and media outlets such as *Parade* magazine, ESPN2, ABC News, CBS News, NBC News, FOX News, the *New York Times* and *Newsweek* magazine, just to name a few. So why all of the attention? I believe it's for the same reason that Curves currently has over 6 million women who swear by their product. We're changing lives for the better—one member at a time.

"In just seven months my husband lost 43 pounds and sparked up the energy that was always within him. He went from an ice cream eating couch potato to an active stallion who enjoys fruits and vegetables. He can work all day and still have energy to do anything . . . I mean anything! He is more playful with the kids and a great role model. He is just as physically fit as he was at 18 years old. Thank you, Cuts, for giving me my high school sweetheart back."

—*Lizette Rivera* on her husband, ALBERTO

Back in 1991, the founder of Curves was smart enough to realize that there was a very large segment of women who were being ignored by the health and fitness industry. Women who would never step foot in a traditional health club because they didn't feel as comfortable exercising there. As our managing director, Steven Haase, often says, the real success behind Curves is explained by the fact that "they loved a large audience of women that had traditionally been unloved by the fitness world." Then, they created a place for these women to go where they could not only exercise, but finally feel accepted for who they were—many, I imagine, for the very first time.

I've had clients find out about Cuts Fitness For Men by word of mouth because we're considered the male equivalent of Curves when it comes to convenient, effective exercise. Others have watched their friends or coworkers transform their physiques using our program and demanded to know how to achieve the same results for themselves. However, the main reason Cuts Fitness For Men has gained worldwide notoriety in such a short time in the fitness industry is obvious.

Most guys may be less inclined to admit it, but I feel the same basic needs apply when it comes to men. We're looking for a place where you're not only shown how to get in shape, but where you can feel a sense of acceptance. It's one of the most important keys to sticking with exercise and making it a habit for life, but it's not the easiest thing to feel as you get older, especially if you've never exercised or thought about leading a healthy lifestyle until now. That's the kind of environment I've tried to create for each and every member of Cuts Fitness. The aim of my clubs has always been to connect with men worldwide at the very deepest level possible, so I could get at the heart of why they don't exercise and finally give them a reason to. I'm proud to say—and the critics agree—that we've done just that.

I'll be honest with you. It's been my experience that most guys have found Cuts Fitness based on their attraction to our 30-minute Body Cuts program workout, a time-efficient, results-proven program that I'll show you later in this book. Time is the number one reason people cite for why they don't exercise. And every time I hear someone say, "I just don't have the time," it makes me angry and upset. "That's right, you don't have the time, which is exactly why you should be exercising!" I fire back, "Did you know that without exercise, you increase your odds of dying prematurely? Did you know that being unhealthy is the fastest way to miss out on many of life's most important events, like watching your kids grow up? Did you know that exercise—no matter how little time you think you have to devote to it—can actually reverse all that, so you not only live a longer life, but you're able to enhance your quality of life starting right now?"

Lack of time may be the main reason our members have turned to Cuts Fitness, but it's finally finding a life-changing plan they can commit to—and stick with—that keeps them walking in our door three times a week. Just like the atmosphere in our clubs, there's no pressure when it comes to all of the exercise tips, tricks and programs you'll learn in this book. All I expect from you is to do what you can for now. The rest will come in time, but the results will start a lot sooner. That promise doesn't just come from me personally, but from thousands of guys just like you who have told us how much our facilities and our programs have changed their lives forever.

Men who were just like you on their very first visit to Cuts Fitness—uncertain of exercise and, more importantly, themselves. I can't tell you how satisfying it is to see these same men just thirty to sixty days later walking around with a newfound sense of confidence and a healthy strut that they either had thought they had lost or had never had before. Ordinary men who came to us leading completely sedentary lifestyles, who not only immediately began to see and feel results, but continue to stick with the Cuts Fitness program. My brother Gary, now fifty-five, has been battling with obesity issues all his life. I have witnessed his pain over the years and have personally experienced the effects that this has had on our family as well. Fortunately, Gary took action and has lost over one hundred pounds over the last year.

He will always be a motivational factor for me as I continue on the path of providing wellness solutions for men around the world. It's that sense of exercise adherence that's the greatest benefit of our program, and it's the reason that once you try our plan—just like all of our members before you—you'll understand why you'll keep coming back.

As a man in my fifties, who has struggled in the past to stay in shape, feel young and hold onto his health, I've been exactly where you are right now.

But I'm not there anymore.

I'm here, enjoying all the rewards that come with finally making the time to follow a healthier lifestyle. I'm at a place in my life where losing the body I once had doesn't have to happen anymore. I'm at a place where feeling good and having plenty of all-day energy is not only possible, it's simply become a natural part of my day. I'm at a place in my life that I never thought I'd ever find time to be.

In short, I'm right at a place where you'll soon be.

If you're ready to go from "there" to "here," the Body Cuts program is more than ready to show you how.

The Body Cuts™ Program: It Started Out of Necessity

Don't look now . . . but your body is conspiring against you.

Did you know that 80 percent of men don't exercise for the recommended three times a week? Even worse, did you know that 60 percent of middle-aged men don't bother to exercise at all? Did you know that half of men in the Western world are overweight, with a startling 13 percent of that number being obese? If I've just described you in any of these statistics, then I have something to share with you.

It doesn't have to be that way.

Getting the physique you've always wanted and changing your life for the better don't have to mean a lot of thinking and tremendous sacrifice. Everything you've ever wanted, from losing that stubborn belly fat, building a better body and, more importantly, lowering your risk of heart disease, diabetes, high blood pressure and all of the major health problems that afflict men today, can start today.

Or, to be more specific, it starts with this book.

Most of the members that step into any of my fitness facilities know me as the president and founder of Cuts Fitness For Men, the world's fastest-growing men's fitness franchise. They also know me as the creator of the Body Cuts program, a comprehensive, thirty-minute circuit training and cardiovascular-based workout designed specifically for men who lack the time—or in some cases, simply the desire—to exercise in a traditional gym. But before all of that, I was—and still am, for that matter—just like you.

Just an older man, looking to reclaim that sense of youth he once had.

I'm fifty-two now, and fortunately, I've managed to stay fit all my life. But that doesn't mean I haven't run into the same obstacles that most men, like yourself, have had to deal with. In fact, it's from those obstacles that my desire to create the Body Cuts Workout was born.

When I first started working in the world of fitness and exercise—back in 1990—I was thirty-six years old. There I was, already considered middle-aged in an industry that not only rewards youth and vitality, it expects it. But staying fit with the hectic career I was about to get into wasn't easy. To be honest, it was a career that truly made it difficult to practice what I was supposed to be preaching. Between all the constant travel, living out of a suitcase and dealing with sixteen-hour days that come from working with clients, exercise—and just watching my own health, for that matter—became the hardest thing to find time for that I had ever dealt with. But being too busy to exercise wasn't the only thing I noticed that getting older was bringing to the table.

Back in my twenties, I didn't just have more time to exercise; I had more energy as well. I could also bounce back from the long workouts I used to do without a single ache or pain. I would spend up to two hours a day at the gym five days a week trying to stay in shape, doing many of the traditional machines and free-weight exercises that were popular at the time. Even on my off days, I'd run on the treadmill for up to an hour, never thinking about how exercise could improve my health and make things easier when I got older. I never thought of how exercising the *right* way could help lower my risk for many of the health problems older men suffer from worldwide on a daily basis. I never thought about how one day, I'd need to follow a more specific workout regime to help me feel, look and be young again. I never thought about much back then. But then again, I never thought those days would stop either.

Then one day, the way I had always exercised—the programs and routines that worked so well in my youth—weren't as effective as they once were. A session of lifting weights the way I used to would bring about a week's worth of aches and pains I wasn't used to. I couldn't bounce back from exercise as quickly anymore, and the results slowed down and eventually stopped altogether.

Suddenly, everything I knew about staying fit seemed worthless to me. Or more to the point, everything I knew about exercise no longer applied to who I was now.

A man that was twice as old as he once was when doing all those exercise programs was a daily part of my life. I had to accept that age was trying to put an end to exercise, if I couldn't figure out a routine that was just as effective, yet even more beneficial, for men looking to turn back time on their bodies.

That's when the Body Cuts program was born.

How to Use This Book

If you're already a Cuts Fitness member, then you're already aware of how effective the program is for helping men reach each and every one of their fitness, health and weight-loss goals. If you're not a member of Cuts Fitness For Men, then don't worry. (It's not a prerequisite, although we'd love to see you in our clubs.) No matter which category you fall in, you'll still use this book in the same exact manner.

This book outlines the Body Cuts workout—the sixteen exercises that have gotten our members in the best shape of their lives. Follow the workout three times a week—or one of the other two versions of the sixteen-station workout in the book that let you perform it at home or on the road—and you're on your way to a healthier new you. However, to accomplish even more results, this book also outlines easy-to-follow Cuts Fitness guidelines you can implement right now when it comes to:

- Eating right
- Eliminating stress
- Watching your overall health
- Getting enough sleep
- Keeping your body flexible and injury-free
- And much more!

The best part about this book is that how much or how little of it you decide to use is entirely up to you. Unlike other diet and exercise books that require you to perform every single step they tell you to do, you *don't* have to do everything I'm about to show you. Just adhering to the Body Cuts workout on a regular three-times-a-week schedule has been enough of a life-changing experience for many of our members. But because this book was designed to go beyond the gym experience, following as many of the Cuts Fitness lifestyle guidelines as possible—depending on what you have time for—can take the traditional Cuts Fitness experience to the next level.

Cuts Success Story #1

Throughout this book, you're going to read testimonials from just a few of the thousands and thousands of Cuts Fitness For Men members worldwide that have used the Body Cuts program and achieved a new lease on their lives, reshaped their bodies and improved their health in ways they never expected. But it all started with Cuts Fitness for Men's very first member.

Me.

Between years spent on the road and hitting my mid to late thirties, all of the issues I had only heard about from older men who were either not exercising, or exercising the wrong way, started becoming my issues as well.

First, it was back pain.

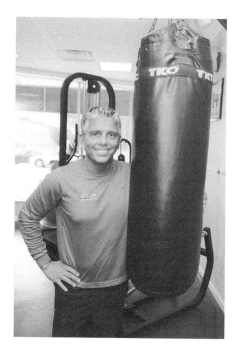

Then, I started losing the energy to work out as often.

Soon, I noticed my muscles starting to shrink.

Before I knew it, I was slowly putting on weight I didn't want in places I didn't expect.

That's when I realized I needed a new exercise program. An exercise program that wasn't as abusive as the workouts of my past, so my body had more time to recover. An exercise program that could help me shed all the unwanted pounds that were beginning to creep in with age and bring back the muscle I once had. An exercise program that was intense enough to get results—yet safe enough to use, no matter how old I was. And finally, an exercise program that I could do in what few minutes I had to devote to exercise each and every week.

The Body Cuts program accomplishes all of that—and so much more, as you'll soon see in yourself. Today, people tell me I look like I'm in my thirties, but to be honest with you, I feel like I'm in my twenties. Physically, I can feel that I'm in better shape now than I was in my teens, when I took my youthful health and body for granted. And when I say "in better shape," I'm not just talking about how much muscle I've regained and how much fat I've been able to lose using the program. Medically, I'm in better control of my health than ever before. More importantly, it's a program that's so easy to fit into my life that I'm finally more in control of it too . . . as are the thousands and thousands of men worldwide that have chosen to use my Body Cuts program.

I may have created the Body Cuts program for myself, but it's my honor to share it with you. So let's get started.

The Five Goals Every Man Should Have

Before I teach you how to make the Body Cuts program a part of your lifestyle, I need to ask you a question: How invested are you *right now* in your health?

That's an odd question to ask, isn't it? After all, you've bought this book, so that should be enough to prove that you're most definitely concerned about your body. But if you truly want to lose weight, get strong, feel energized and regain your youth, it's a very serious question that demands a very serious answer.

Of the thousands and thousands of men I've met over the years while demonstrating and explaining Cuts Fitness For Men and my Body Cuts program, I've met a lot who thought they were on the right path to better health and a better body, but I've only met a handful that were truly invested in their health before starting the plan.

Cuts SUCCESS STORY 214

"It fits right in with my lifestyle."

KURT LIBBY   AGE: 63   Alameda, CA

"Throughout my life, I had always been pretty athletic, which is why it was so hard to accept that I wasn't in shape anymore as I got older. It was when I finally admitted to myself that I was getting fat in all the areas that I had once been fit that made me decide enough was enough. I wasn't interested in trying to develop my own workout, so I turned to Cuts. [The Body Cuts program] works right in with my day with minimal disruption to my life. Thanks, John!"

Oh sure, each member of Cuts Fitness would soon learn how to become fully vested in taking control of his health, his heart and his physique using the Body Cuts program. But on that very day they decided to finally take fitness seriously, most members had the will to get in shape but were unfortunately clueless about a few key factors that would ultimately decide whether they saw every positive result they expect.

How could I know this? Easy.

I've discovered that by having the clients of my gym be truthful about five specific things, I can assess whether or not they're already on the right path to a better life. That's right. It all comes down to five very simple—yet very important—personal goals that every man should strive for throughout his life. For men, just reaching even *one* of these five goals is a serious step in the right direction. But when all five are in place, you can significantly reduce your body fat, build lean muscle where you need it most and improve your health a thousandfold.

Here are the five most important goals every guy should strive for and be able to say yes to (in no particular order of importance, because believe me, each is just as vital as the rest) and why they are so important for men.

THE FIVE MOST IMPORTANT GOALS
EVERY MAN BETTER SAY YES TO

- I strength train for at least 30 minutes a day, three times a week.
- I know what my "maximum heart rate" is.
- My waist is around the same size as my hips.
- I get at least eight hours of sleep a night.
- I visit a doctor as often as I should.

I STRENGTH TRAIN FOR AT LEAST 30 MINUTES A DAY, THREE TIMES A WEEK

When you really step back and look at this first goal compared to the other four, it's probably one of the easiest to reach. But is it one that you can *honestly* say you do on a weekly basis?

Performing some sort of strength training regime for at least twenty minutes, three times a week is what nearly all experts in the exercise and fitness industry recommend that men—no matter what their age—do each and every week. When you add it up—twenty minutes, three times a week—that's only one hour of your time for the week.

Now I want you to try out a few other math problems for me. Try adding up how much time you spend each week waiting in line. Now add up how long it takes you to commute to work. How about the number of hours each week you spend watching sports? Reading the paper? Killing time on the toilet, perhaps? I'm a betting man, and I'm willing to wager that all of those totals are longer than one hour a week. Am I right? Only you know the answer. But here's why taking one hour away from all the nonproductive activities you typically do each week, to strength train instead—using the Body Cuts program—is such an essential goal that you—or your body—simply can't ignore it any longer.

Strength Training: Why It's Especially Important for Men

Most older guys already know that regular strength training is the perfect recipe for building and maintaining lean muscle tissue. Whether you used to weight train when you were younger, tried in the past but were never happy with the results or are just thinking about doing it for the first time by picking up this book, chances are you're already aware that it's the first step toward reshaping your physique into a younger-looking body that's more powerful and more attractive.

However, the benefits of strength training go far beyond just improving your appearance on the outside. Here's why this particular goal should always be a top priority on every older guy's to-do list:

It prevents you from replacing muscle with fat

Does the scale confuse you sometimes? You step on it, only to find out you still weigh the same as you did a few years ago. There's only one problem.

Why don't you look as good as you used to a few years ago?

Most men don't realize that after age thirty, their body sheds a half pound of muscle each year. That may not seem that important, but research has shown that your body spends an additional thirty-five to forty-five calories each day just to maintain every pound of muscle you have. Losing that little bit of muscle leaves your body no choice but to store those extra twelve hundred calories every month as unwanted body fat.

That's why if you don't strength train, you could be replacing a half pound of muscle with a half pound of new fat, even though your scale may still say you weigh the same. The easiest way to stop this change from happening is to use strength training to replace the muscle that age is trying to take away. That's where your first goal comes into play.

Studies have shown that two months of strength training, performed two or three times a week for twenty minutes, can replace three pounds of fat with three pounds of muscle. You may not see a difference on the scale, but adding that extra muscle helps you burn an extra 120 calories a day just to maintain it, extra calories that otherwise would have added to your waistline and other places you would rather not think about.

It reduces your risk of injury

Not only does regular strength training improve your balance and coordination so you're less likely to be accident-prone, it also restores the density of your bones. Throughout your life, your bone tissue consistently breaks down and replaces itself naturally. But after you turn thirty-five, that process slows down, causing your bones to break down more quickly than they can add new bone mass. What that can lead to is a condition most men think they're immune to—osteoporosis. However, men are just as susceptible to developing this condition, especially if they aren't taking the right steps to prevent it.

Regular strength training can reverse that deterioration by making your bones grow just as much as your muscles. How does it do that? As you strength train, your body responds by increasing the amount of bone mineral composition, which in turn helps your bones become strong enough to handle the stress placed on them through exercise. The end result: thicker, healthier bones that are not only less brittle, but more resilient to any snaps or breaks that life may have in store for you later.

"I did it to keep looking good for my wife."

KEN HERMAN AGE: 47 Levittown, PA

"Every guy has the same amount of time to spend on exercise, but for me, I just didn't have the time to work out anymore. I was in a rut, working too much and finding myself buying larger pants every few years. Finally, I looked at my wife—who is gorgeous—and decided I had to do something. I've been using the [Body Cuts program] for over a year now and it definitely gives me maximum results for the time I have to spend."

It decreases—and increases—your cholesterol

Did you know that the levels of cholesterol in your body rise with age? It's a fact that puts many older men at risk of developing heart disease each and every year. That's where regular strength training can even the odds in your favor. According to a *Journal of Gerontology* study, resistance training may improve cholesterol levels by decreasing LDL levels in your body—the "bad" cholesterol that can build up along your arteries, block blood flow and increase your risk of heart disease—while it simultaneously increases the amount of HDL cholesterol in your system—the "good" kind that draws cholesterol away from your arteries and back to your liver, where your body has an easier time removing it from your system.

It reduces your risk of diabetes

According to the National Institute of Diabetes and Digestive and Kidney Disease, over 8.7 million—or 8.7 percent of all men over the age of twenty in the United States—have diabetes. So how does strength training have any effect on this growing problem? With type II diabetes, your body either doesn't produce enough insulin to help regulate your blood sugar (otherwise known as glucose) or your cells just ignore insulin in your system altogether. When you add exercise to the equation, your body uses less insulin to transport glucose into your cells, which helps regulate your blood sugar. The result can have a substantial effect on preventing and/or improving type I and type II diabetes.

It can lessen your daily aches and pains

A lot of people associate exercise with feeling achy, but regular strength training can actually lessen all the stiffness and pains that make a man *feel* far older than he really is. In fact, it could save you money down the road by reducing your need for over-the-counter (and under-the-counter) pain medications and prescriptions. A study performed at Tufts University examined the effects of a sixteen-week strength-training program on older individuals with moderate to severe knee osteoarthritis. What they discovered was that strength training was just as effective—if not more effective—than the medications they were using to decrease their pain. Subjects had decreased their pain by as much as 43 percent, all through a steady regime of routine strength training.

I KNOW WHAT MY "MAXIMUM HEART RATE" IS

If you've achieved this goal, it means that you at least know what "maximum heart rate" means—or MHR, as it's sometimes called. That's the maximum number of contractions per minute—otherwise known as beats—that your heart can make. The older you get, the more your MHR slows down, which means your heart naturally begins to slow down. If you have no idea what your MHR is, here's how to figure out that number on your own.

"I've lost one-fifth of my body weight, thanks to the Body Cuts program."

RICHARD LEES AGE: 64 Clifton, NJ

"My weight before trying the Body Cuts program for men was 237 pounds, which is why I joined originally for health reasons. Even though I was obese and on medication for having high blood pressure, I still found it hard to devote myself to regular exercise because most gyms were too 'macho' and intimidating. To be honest, I couldn't even find the time even in my own home. But with the Body Cuts program, I finally found a system that works for me. Today, my blood pressure medication has been halved by my doctor, in part due to all the weight loss so far. Thanks for making exercise comfortable again, John."

To find out your maximum heart rate, just subtract your age from the number 220. That means if you're forty-five years old, your maximum heart rate is 220 minus 45 (or 175 beats per minute). If you hate math, I've done a few examples already for you:

- If you're 25, your MHR would be 195.
- If you're 30, your MHR would be 190.
- If you're 35, your MHR would be 185.
- If you're 40, your MHR would be 180.
- If you're 45, your MHR would be 175.
- If you're 50, your MHR would be 170.
- If you're 55, your MHR would be 165.
- If you're 60, your MHR would be 160.
- If you're 65, your MHR would be 155.
- If you're 70, your MHR would be 150.
- If you're 75, your MHR would be 145.
- If you're 80, your MHR would be 140.

So what exactly is this number and why is knowing it so important to me—or, should I say, important to you? You see, I've found that those men that know their MHR usually end up already knowing a little something about cardiovascular exercise and its many health benefits. That's because in order to do cardiovascular exercise correctly and safely, this one, single number is the best way to judge if you're underworking—or overworking—your heart.

Most experts recommend that men do some form of moderate-intensity cardio-vascular exercise for at least 30 minutes a day, three days a week. But just because you break a sweat doesn't always mean you're exercising hard enough to reap any benefits—especially if your goal is to burn off excess fat. To do that, you have to exercise hard enough to elevate your heart rate and maintain your pulse at a certain amount of your maximum heart rate—typically 60 to 70 percent of your MHR.

For example, if you're forty-five years old, then you already know your MHR is 175.

- 60% of 175 would be 105 beats per minute (bpm)
- 70% of 175 would be 122 beats per minute (bpm)

That means that if you're a forty-five-year-old man, the best way to burn fat is by doing some sort of physical activity that keeps your heart rate between 105 and 122 beats per minute, three times a week. So what exactly happens if your pulse is higher or lower than that as you exercise? Well, as I'll discuss in Chapter 9, there are different benefits—as well as health risks—to either elevating your pulse any higher or keeping it lower than 60 to 70 percent of your MHR. But to see the most effective—and safest—results, I prefer that you keep your pulse in this particular zone—which I call the "Fat Burning Zone."

Here is how the numbers break down:

AGE	MHR	FAT BURNING ZONE (60–70%)
25	195	117 up to 136 bpm
30	190	114 up to 133 bpm
35	185	111 up to 129 bpm
40	180	108 up to 126 bpm
45	175	105 up to 122 bpm
50	170	102 up to 119 bpm
55	165	99 up to 115 bpm
60	160	96 up to 112 bpm
65	155	93 up to 108 bpm
70	150	90 up to 105 bpm
75	145	87 up to 101 bpm
80	140	84 up to 98 bpm

Cardiovascular Exercise: Why It's Especially Important for Men

I mentioned earlier in this chapter that your body loses muscle as you age, but there's something else that starts to fade as well. Your metabolism—the number of calories your body burns to remain functional throughout the day—begins to slow down around age thirty. This "metabolic slowdown" causes your body to use fewer calories throughout the day, which means your body gets stuck with more and more unused calories, which it has no choice but to convert into excess body fat. That's why, on average, most men begin to gain one pound of fat every year from this metabolism downshift.

Cardiovascular exercise—also known as "cardio" or "aerobic" exercise—can change all that. The term "cardiovascular exercise" may sound scientific, but it really refers to any activity that makes your heart beat faster and lungs breathe harder for a certain period of time. Adding cardiovascular exercise to your plan can burn off those leftover calories before they ever have the chance to turn into fat, but it also does a lot more for your body than just control and reduce the amount of fat you store.

Regular cardiovascular exercise also improves your level of fitness by training the heart and lungs to be more effective in delivering oxygen. By making your heart muscles stronger through cardiovascular exercise, you make it easier for them to do their job of delivering more oxygen-rich blood throughout your body. The end result for you: more oxygen in your system to use as energy and an increase in the good cholesterol (HDL) in your system (which has been shown to reduce the risk of heart disease). In fact, your risk of everything from high blood pressure and stroke, to diabetes and certain types of cancers, such as colon cancer and breast cancer, all decrease the sooner you start doing some form of regular cardiovascular exercise—and staying within the right aerobic zone by using your MHR as your guide.

Find Your Pulse—Instantly

UNLIKE OTHER GYMS or clubs that leave it up to you to bring whatever's necessary to monitor your pulse, many of our Cuts Fitness For Men facilities have mini heart rate monitors between exercise stations. But figuring out your pulse without any help is easy. Here's how:

- Stop in the middle of whatever physical activity you're doing.
- Place two fingers—your index and middle finger—along the side of your neck or on the top of your wrist.
- Press down slightly until you can feel your pulse.
- Start counting how many times your heart beats in six seconds. Start the count on a beat—which you'll count as zero.
- Take that number and times it by ten—or just add a zero to the end of the number. (The number you're left with is your beats per minute, or bpm.)
- Check to see if that number falls somewhere between the "zone" you should be in. If it's lower, try exercising at a brisker pace; if it's higher, slow down and/or take a rest if you're overexerting yourself.

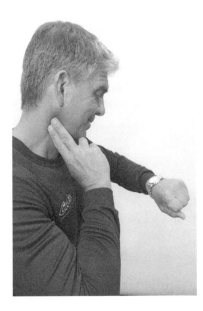

MY WAIST IS AROUND THE SAME SIZE AS MY HIPS

If I asked you how big your arms were, I have a feeling you would be more than happy to roll up your sleeve, grab the tape measure and flex proudly. But if I asked you how big your butt was, you'd probably want to leave me flat on mine just for inquiring.

But here's a secret most men aren't aware of. Knowing how big—or small—your butt is in relation to your belly is one of the most important measurements you'll ever take in your life. I know it sounds like a female thing, but I'm not asking you to measure it for vanity sake. It's because that specific measurement is the key to knowing how susceptible you are to many of the health issues that men face as they get older. The good news is that it's also the key to lowering your risk as well.

Now that I have your attention, let's see where you stack up before I continue. I need you to be your own personal tailor for two important measurements. Don't worry—no one needs to know you're taking these measurements but you and me. Here's what I want you to do:

- First, just stand straight with your best posture—that means with a flat back and your head held high as if you're at attention—if you want the most accurate measurement. Remember, you're only cheating yourself if you try to "skew" what the tape tells you.
- Next, holding this posture, take a measurement around your hips. Wrap it straight around the widest part of your hips—again, trying to fudge the numbers will keep these numbers from helping your health. To help you determine the widest part of your hips, try doing this measurement in front of a mirror, or measure your hips several times (lowering the tape an inch each time) and take the highest number out of all the measurements.
- Next, measure your waist using the same strategy—either with a mirror, or take several measurements and choose the widest. Don't suck in your belly; again, you're only cheating your health if you do. This isn't about your looks; it's about your life.
- Finally, divide your waist measurement by your hip measurement. For example, if your waist is 38 inches and your hips are 42 inches, then you would divide 38 by 42 and end up with .9 as your final number.

It's this final number that can give you an instant assessment if your health may be at risk. Doctors agree that you want to try and maintain a number of .9 or lower. For both men and women, having a waist-hip ratio that's 1.0 or higher means you're more likely to be considered overweight for your height. It also means you might be more at risk of developing a multitude of undesirable health issues. Research has shown that guys with more weight around their waists face more health risks (from diabetes and certain types of cancer to the number one killer of men, heart disease) than men who carry more weight around their hips instead.

Cuts SUCCESS STORY 481

"I've lost the fat and gained back my energy."

MELVIN FOSTER AGE: 37 Dover, PA

"My new line of work as a pastor made me less active, but I still wanted to lose my gut and gain back energy. I knew I needed to exercise, but I don't like the atmosphere of most gyms, plus, I also felt that most gyms take up too much time. The atmosphere of Cuts is great, the [Body Cuts] program encourages you along the way, and the fact that it only takes 30 minutes a day makes it quick and enjoyable."

A Smaller Waistline: Why It's Especially Important for Men

It's hard to say yes to this goal when your ever-growing waistline has other plans, right? But there's a reason for that. Many men never adjust to how their metabolism begins to slow with age, and they continue consuming the same number of calories they did when their metabolism ran much faster. Eventually, all those extra calories catch up to your belly.

Every extra pound you're carrying around your middle—and elsewhere, for that matter—does more than cause a health risk, it makes you more tired than you should be. Fat tissue still requires a constant source of blood in order to stay functional. With only so much blood to go around, this extra demand for it from excess belly fat ends up thinning out the amount of oxygen distributed to the rest of the body. At the same time, the extra weight of belly fat simultaneously taxes your cardiovascular system by making your heart work harder every minute of the day. The combination of the two can be a drain on your energy all day long, even when you're simply standing still.

I GET AT LEAST EIGHT HOURS OF SLEEP A NIGHT

Unlike the other three goals, which take some amount of work to achieve, this fourth one should be the easiest of the bunch to pull off, right? But for something as easy as putting down your head and passing out for one-third of the day, a surprising 70 million people suffer from some sort of sleeping disorder in the United States alone, according to the U.S. Institute of Health.

Whether you find yourself staying up watching late-night television, waiting for your kids to get home or worrying about your 401(k), burning the midnight oil can have more of a negative impact on your physical and emotional health than most guys realize. In fact, research has shown that not taking this goal seriously and depriving yourself of sleep can negatively affect almost every aspect of how your body functions.

It can impair your memory. It can boost your risk of high blood pressure. It's even been shown to shorten your life span, according to a study performed at Harvard Medical School that found that sleeping less than six hours a night had a significant impact on people's overall mortality. But if lack of sleep's effect on your health doesn't bother you, let me explain how not reaching this goal may also be aging the way you look.

Quality Sleep: Why It's Especially Important for Men

The average guy needs seven to eight hours of sleep a night. Unfortunately, many men typically get less, about an hour less than that. That one-hour loss can have more of an effect on you than just a set of saggy eyes. It can leave your muscles looking saggier as well.

Not getting enough sleep regularly can cause your body's level of HGH (human growth hormone)—a hormone produced by the pituitary gland that stimulates the growth of muscle, cartilage and bone tissue—to drop significantly on a daily basis. With less HGH in your system, your muscles are left with less to grow from. Getting enough sleep can prevent that daily drop in HGH from ever happening.

Being sleep deprived also causes your body to actually burn away the muscles you've worked so hard to rebuild. How does it do that? Your immune system needs time to rest in order to heal itself after you work out, but getting less sleep than you need leaves your body very little energy to repair itself later on. Being overly tired also raises your body's production of adrenaline—a hormone that helps your body deal with stress. The two problems combined place your body in a higher catabolic state, causing it to cannibalize its own muscle tissue to use for energy. That can leave your body with even fewer results to show for all your efforts at exercise.

"I get twice the results in one simple plan."

RON SAMA AGE: 47 Forked River, NJ

"I was looking for a workout to look better and feel healthier as I get older. What I got with Cuts Fitness went beyond that. I enjoy getting amazing physical results from a routine that doesn't just improve my muscles, but my heart as well. The way this 30-minute routine combines aerobic training with anaerobic training in the shortest time possible has me in better shape than guys half my age. I couldn't have done it without the Body Cuts program."

I VISIT A DOCTOR AS OFTEN AS I SHOULD

If this last goal is one you can honestly say you stick to, then I'm proud of you. But on average, older guys like us are statistically the worst demographic when it comes to seeing a doctor as often as we should.

Unless you already have a health condition that concerns your doctor, most experts agree on the following guidelines on how often men should have a checkup.

- Teenage years to 30: See a doctor twice in your twenties.
- 30–65: Every 1–2 years—or as often as your doctor recommends.
- Over 65: Every year—or as often as your doctor recommends.

So where do you rank? And if you thought you were seeing your doctor often enough, are you still achieving your goal, now that you're more aware of how often you should be going for a checkup? If not, like I said before, you're definitely not alone.

One of the main reasons most men avoid seeing a physician is because they're simply afraid to hear any bad news pertaining to their health. But that kind of logic can actually bring on bad news. Many of the health issues that affect us older men over the years can actually start showing up in our late teens and early twenties. Getting out of the habit of "dodging the doc" can keep you living well beyond your years, if you're smart enough to make it a goal you'll stick with for a lifetime. That's why later on, in Chapter 8, I'm going to teach you all you need to know about what to expect from a doctor's visit—and how to make the most of it. But for now, here's why I need you to make those trips a regular part of your routine.

Regular Checkups: Why They're Especially Important for Men

Hypertension, diabetes, cancer and most major diseases that affect men are serious issues that almost never make themselves known until it's too late to do anything about them. Letting a physician do his or her job every once in a while can help you spot these problems at their earliest stages, when they are most likely to be treated, prevented or cured.

TWO

THE COMPLETE CUTS FITNESS FOR MEN WORKOUT

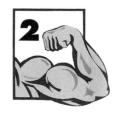

THE BODY CUTS™ PROGRAM

THE SECRET TO REACHING ALL FIVE GOALS

So . . . where exactly did you rank?

If you said yes to all five goals, many experts and doctors agree that you could have the body you deserve and add an additional ten years to your life. However, if you said no to all five, then unfortunately, those same experts and doctors expect it could mean the exact opposite. Not paying attention to all five goals doesn't just shorten your life span; it can make you lead the life you're left with running on less energy, poor health and a body that looks older than it really is.

But here's the good news. Or should I say, here's the great news.

It doesn't matter whether you could honestly check off one, two, three or four of the five goals on my list. Quite frankly, it doesn't even matter if you couldn't even check off one. And if you were able to check off all five with pride, I still have great news for you too. In fact, because you already know how much hard work and patience it takes to achieve all five goals and make them part of your life, you'll appreciate what I have to say that much more.

The 30-minute Body Cuts program is designed to help you reach—and maintain—the five most important goals that every man should achieve, quickly, effectively and, best of all, simultaneously.

You'll strength train three times a week

The muscle you lose as you age isn't so much from losing on a cellular level, but from having your muscle cells atrophy—or shrink—from inactivity. The Body Cuts program is an easy-to-use, full-body plan that makes it fun to get in the required three days a week of strength training your body needs to "reinflate" your muscle cells and bring back the muscle you once had when you were younger.

You'll know your MHR and always use it to your advantage

The Body Cuts program uses a series of exercises that—when done as a circuit—raise your heart rate to the same elevated levels as cardiovascular exercise. Unlike other workouts that have you train your muscles with strength training, then train your heart afterward with cardiovascular exercise, the Body Cuts program combines both into one muscle-building, heart-healthy cardiovascular plan.

"I haven't had this much energy in years."

KEVIN KAVANAUGH AGE: 51 Ewing, NJ

"I try to stay in shape by kayaking three times a week from May to October, but how often I could do it always depends on my energy. Thanks to Cuts, I have more energy, more flexibility and my cholesterol dropped from 278 to 220. But my results don't stop there. Soon after using the Body Cuts program, I found myself with enough energy to dance for three hours straight two nights in a row . . . and, I even did the twist all the way to the floor. I was even recently told that I look 38, but the best part is that I feel 28. Thanks for making it easy, John."

You'll improve your sleep dramatically

The Body Cuts program is the perfect prescription for a better night's sleep. Research has shown that regular exercise places stress on the body that forces your brain to compensate by increasing its need for deep sleep. The mix of exercises you'll be using in all three Cuts Fitness workouts in this book challenge and strengthen larger muscle groups—the legs, chest and back—which helps even further to bring about the level of fatigue needed to let you sleep faster and more soundly. Think of it as the ideal trade-off for your body: thirty minutes of work for a full eight hours of quality sleep that will not only leave you more refreshed, but looking—and feeling—healthier.

You'll lose fat from everywhere—especially your belly

The intensity of the Body Cuts program is unlike other strength-training programs you might have tried in the past. Instead of wasting time between exercises, you move from one exercise to the next, which doesn't just exercise your heart—as I just mentioned—but forces your body to burn even more calories while you work out.

You'll hear only good news from your doctor

How can the Body Cuts program get you to go to the doctor more often? Simple. By ensuring that all you ever hear from your doctor is nothing but compliments about how well you're taking care of yourself. That's because keeping your body fat low and your heart healthy through regular exercise can help prevent many of the major health problems most men suffer from, before they start. But what the Body Cuts program offers you goes beyond that.

Did you know that research has shown that men who expended two thousand calories per week had an increased life expectancy of two years? Studies have proven that a single hour of exercise can extend your life span by two hours. The Body Cuts program is a 30-minute-a-day, three-times-a-week plan. That means for every week you use and stay dedicated to the Body Cuts program in this book, you'll be adding an additional three hours a week to your life.

Why the Cuts Fitness For Men Program Works

When I first designed the official sixteen-station circuit that would become the Body Cuts program back in 2003, it had to help men reach all of the goals I mentioned—which I hope are now your goals as well. I started by experimenting with a modified circuit of exercises that had been used for many years, especially by the military. But because I didn't have two hours to spend exercising like in the past—all I had was 30 minutes tops—the program had to accomplish the same results in one-quarter of the time.

However, it also had to encompass the most fundamental elements that a workout needs to have to be as effective as possible.

What Every Successful Workout Should Do

Once you're ready to incorporate strength training into your life, the key to getting the best results in the quickest amount of time is making the most of every single workout. To do that, there are several tried-and-true, scientifically proven, no-fail fitness tips that every workout program should have:

1. **It should be a full-body affair.** It's important to make sure any strength training routine you start works all the major—and minor—muscles in your body. It should always include exercises that work all of the following muscle groups: legs, chest, shoulders, back, biceps, triceps and, most important, the core muscles within the lower back and abdominal region.

2. **It should always use a mix of compound exercises.** Picking compound moves—which are exercises that work several muscle groups together, such as squats, chest and shoulder presses, etc.—can make your gym time more productive, giving your body double the results in half the time. Many novice exercisers tend to use exercises that focus strictly on one muscle at a time. These type of exercises—known as isolation exercises—are effective, but they don't teach your muscles to work with one another as they do in everyday life.

3. **It should always force you to do three sets of any exercise.** Performing three sets of the same exercise—which simply means performing the exercise three times in the same workout—is considered the magic number when exercising. Why? Research has shown that repeating an exercise three times helps the muscles you're trying to improve develop more thoroughly.

4. **You should never waste too much time between exercises.** After each set, your muscles need a chance to build their strength back up in order to perform that same exercise again. Generally, thirty to sixty seconds is enough, but most men tend to linger between exercises a lot longer. The problem: if you rest for too long between exercises, you give your muscles time to cool down. That can leave them more prone to injury once you finally continue on with the rest of your workout.

5. **You should always take a day off between workouts.** Muscles don't grow during your workout, they actually grow while you're resting in between your workouts. You see, a good workout not only breaks down your muscles, it also lets them know how you expect them to grow and change. After that, they need time to repair themselves to be ready for the next time. This "muscle remodeling" only takes place when your muscles are left to

rest for at least forty-eight hours. That's why the best exercise programs are ones that are designed to give your muscles enough time in between workouts to heal and grow.

"I got my confidence back, courtesy of Cuts."

STEVE NASH AGE: 42 Glendora, CA

"I once had a job that kept me on my feet all day long for years and years, so I always seemed to stay in shape. But after a career change, I took a job where sitting down for most of the time was the norm. I needed a new way to exercise, but a divorce took a lot of my confidence away from me. After meeting the woman of my dreams—who happens to be a nurse—I knew I had to finally refocus on my health. Cuts offers me a pleasant environment to exercise in and get in shape, but best of all, I enjoy the camaraderie I get from exercising with other guys that are in the same exact situation. Now, between my career, love life and my new shape (20 pounds gone so far), I have never been happier."

If these five tips are too much for you to think about, I'm right there with you. That's why when I designed the Body Cuts program, I crafted it to make things even easier for the average older guy. I know you don't have the time to worry about whether or not the exercise routine you're doing incorporates all five of these elements. You're probably just lucky that you've found the time within your busy schedule. That's why the Body Cuts 30-minute, three-days-a-week program automatically builds these additional elements into your workout.

How exactly can it possibly accomplish that?

1. **All three versions of the Body Cuts program** in this book—the health club version I've just shown you, the at-home version and the on-the-road version—each uses a mix of moves that stress every major muscle group within your body, so you're guaranteed to get a full-body workout each and every time.

2. **Many of the exercises that have been selected** for the Body Cuts program are compound movements that work several muscles at once. To give the

did you know that . . .
Checking off each workout you successfully finish on a calendar can keep you from missing future workouts? Studies have shown that seeing physical proof of your accomplishments makes it easier to motivate yourself at a later date. After every workout, mark it on your day planner and watch how much easier it is to stay the course.

workout even more of an edge, some of the exercises also force you to move not just one type of joint at a time—hip, knee, shoulder, elbow, etc.—but several types of joints at the same time. For example, you'll perform squats (which activate both the hip and knee joints simultaneously) and certain rows and pressing moves (which activate the shoulder and elbow joints at the same time). These type of multijoint exercises require more energy than regular single-joint exercises, helping you burn additional calories while evoking a greater release of muscle-building and fat-burning hormones.

3. **The Body Cuts program is a sixteen-station circuit** of exercises that you'll perform one after the next. However, because you repeat the circuit of exercises three times total, you end up doing exactly three sets of each exercise. The added advantage to the Body Cuts program is that it forces you to give your all to each and every set. When most guys do an exercise in the traditional way—doing three sets before moving onto the next exercise—they usually save up their strength for their third and final set, making their first two sets nothing more than a warm-up. By jumping from station to station, you end up pushing yourself as hard as possible with each set, making each of the three sets as efficient as the others.

4. **There's no wasting a single second in the Body Cuts program.** The sixteen-station circuit is arranged so that you alternate between exercises that work upper-body muscles (the muscles above the waist, such as your chest, back and arms) and exercises that work lower-body muscles (such as your hamstrings, quadriceps and calves). This lets your lower body rest while your upper body is working, and vice versa, allowing you to work your muscles intensely with very little downtime between sets, for a faster, more effective workout.

5. **With the Body Cuts program, you train every muscle** in your body in one session. Not only does that let you enjoy more time away from exercise, but it also lets you space out your workouts every other day. By using the program Mondays, Wednesdays and Fridays, for example, you automatically get one day of rest between each workout to give your muscles enough time to rebuild and grow.

AT THE GYM

THE OFFICIAL BODY CUTS™ WORKOUT

Note: Some Cuts facilities will feature slight variations
in equipment and order of exercises.

The Body Cuts workout is the first 30-minute cardiovascular-/muscle-training program for men that's specially designed to crunch a normal two-hour workout into a safe, effective 30-minute routine.

The official Body Cuts workout available in our facilities is a mix of sixteen different exercise machines—or stations—that, when put together, create a unique full-body workout that strengthens your heart and muscles while it burns off body fat. To perform it, you simply walk in (as a member, of course) and start exercising by sitting down at any of the sixteen stations that aren't being used.

"Cuts has given him something to look forward to in the mornings, given him a healthier future and one hell of a sexier body!"

—Irene Lees on her husband, RICHARD

Once you start the exercise, you continue to do as many repetitions as you can for a total of forty seconds. After that, you are prompted by a recorded voice to move to the next station. Once you reach the end of the circuit, you're instructed to check your pulse to make sure you're exercising within your target heart rate zone. If your pulse is lower than your target zone, you'll increase the intensity of your workout or raise the amount of weight you're using with each exercise; if it's higher than your target heart rate, you will rest until your pulse falls back down in your target zone, then try exercising at a lower intensity when you repeat the circuit.

Repeating the sixteen-station circuit three times only takes approximately 30 minutes, giving you a total-body, fat-burning workout that's not only time-efficient, but strengthens and tones your body from head to toe. Plus, because it forces you to move quickly from station to station, members find that they push themselves much harder than they might do alone at home using standard workout routines—or in clubs that don't give their clients the attention they deserve.

You'll end your workout in the stretching area, where you'll learn how to loosen up all the muscles you've just worked, to keep them flexible and pain-free. Because of the program's unique design, the risk of getting hurt at any age or fitness level is very low.

Cuts
SUCCESS STORY
2,365

"Get off your butt with Cuts."

CLIF PARKER AGE: 83 Newport News, VA

"My biggest problem with getting in shape was simply being inactive. I really needed to slim down and become more active because of my age. But after I signed on the dotted line with Cuts Fitness, I knew I was going to get what I paid for. The Body Cuts program forced me to keep at it."

Before exercising, warm up your muscles
with 3–5 minutes of a low-intensity
cardiovascular exercise, either by jumping in place
or briskly walking around your room.

Maximize the Body Cuts™ Workout

TO GET THE most from every move in the program and to stay injury-free along the way, here are a few important rules you should follow when using this workout—and the other workouts in this book:

- Whenever possible, warm up your muscles before each workout with three to five minutes of a light cardiovascular exercise, such as brisk walking or just walking in place. When you raise the temperature of a muscle, you decrease the risk of injury by making the muscle more pliable. Warming up beforehand also gives you more flexibility, for a greater range of motion, and helps to minimize muscle soreness afterward.
- Do each exercise slowly and smoothly to start. The best rhythm is to raise the weight for a count of two and lower the weight for a count of four. Taking twice as long to lower the weight guarantees that you won't let gravity do the work instead of the muscles you're trying to reshape.
- Never lock your joints as you straighten your arms and legs. Locking out your elbows and/or knees takes the emphasis of the exercise off of your muscles and places additional stress on your joints instead.
- Don't forget to breathe. A lot of men make the mistake of holding their breath as they lift. That's a big mistake for two reasons. First, it raises your blood pressure, but it also cuts off valuable oxygen your body needs for energy. Instead, breath continuously throughout each exercise, exhaling as you lift the weight and inhaling as you lower it.
- Listen to your body. If you feel any pain, stop immediately. You should only experience soreness in the muscles you're trying to work.

THE OFFICIAL
BODY CUTS™ WORKOUT

Exercise		How to Do It
1	Chest Press	Perform for 40 seconds; move on to station #2.
2	Hydraulic Stepper	Perform for 40 seconds; move on to station #3.
3	Pec Contractor	Perform for 40 seconds; move on to station #4.
4	Leg Extension	Perform for 40 seconds; move on to station #5.
5	Triceps Pulldown	Perform for 40 seconds; move on to station #6.
6	Vertical Knee Raise	Perform for 40 seconds; move on to station #7.
7	Spin Bike	Perform for 40 seconds; move on to station #8.
8	Leg Press	Perform for 40 seconds; move on to station #9.
9	Breeze Bike	Perform for 40 seconds; move on to station #10.
10	Seated Abdominal Crunch	Perform for 40 seconds; move on to station #11.
11	Lat Pulldown	Perform for 40 seconds; move on to station #12.
12	Hydraulic Stepper	Perform for 40 seconds; move on to station #13.
13	Cable Curl	Perform for 40 seconds; move on to station #14.
14	Shoulder Press	Perform for 40 seconds; move on to station #15.
15	Ab Slant Decline Bench	Perform for 40 seconds; move on to station #16.
16	Rowing Machine	Perform for 40 seconds; start the cycle over again by starting again with station #1. Repeat the cycle 3 times total.

CHEST PRESS

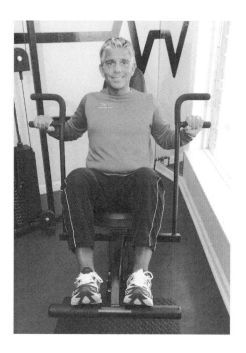 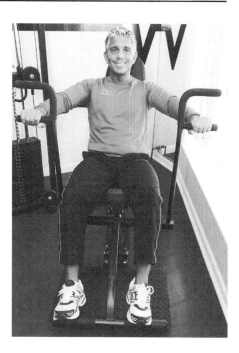

MUSCLES USED: CHEST, SHOULDERS AND TRICEPS

Here's how to do it:

1. Sit on the bench with your feet flat on the floor—or resting on the bottom bar of the machine.
2. Sit back far enough so that your body is flush with the bench from your head to your butt.
3. Grab the handles with both hands and you're ready to begin.
4. Keeping your back flat, push the handles out away from you until your arms are straight, elbows unlocked.
5. Slowly lower the bar back down until it touches your chest—if it doesn't, just lower it as far as you can—and repeat.

   Continue the exercise for a total of 40 seconds, then move on to station #2.

HYDRAULIC STEPPER

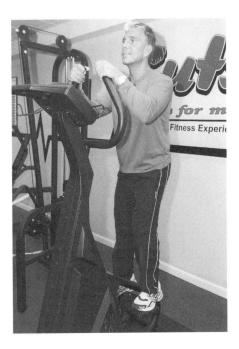

MUSCLES USED: LEGS

Here's how to do it:

1. Step up onto the machine and place your feet flat on the foot pedals.
2. Grab the handles at your sides for support, then begin stepping. The action should feel as though you are walking up a flight of steps.

Continue the exercise for a total of 40 seconds, then move on to station #3.

PEC CONTRACTOR

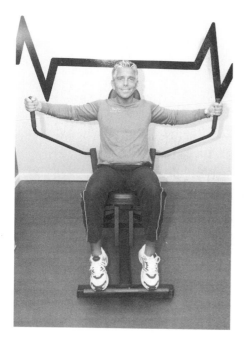 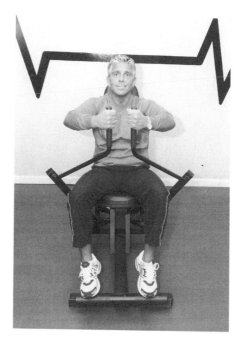

MUSCLES USED: CHEST AND SHOULDERS

Here's how to do it:

1. Sit on the machine and reach out to your sides to grab the handles—your palms should face forward; your arms should be slightly bent, with your elbows pointing down.

2. Keeping your back flat against the bench, sweep your arms in front of you in a semicircular motion until your hands come together in front of your body. (Imagine you're trying to wrap your arms around a large tree.) Squeeze your chest muscles for a second to contract your muscles.

3. Lower your arms back out to your sides and repeat.

Continue the exercise for a total of 40 seconds, then move on to station #4.

LEG EXTENSION

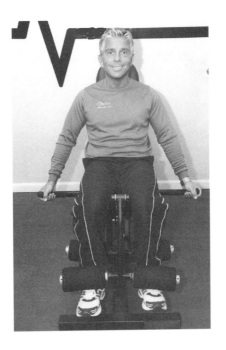 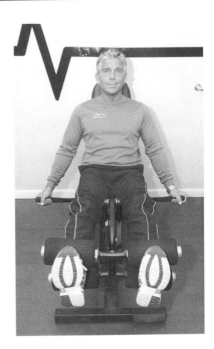

MUSCLES USED: QUADRICEPS

Here's how to do it:

1. Sit down in the seat and hook both feet underneath the padded bar by your ankles.
2. Adjust the pad and/or the seat so that your knees hang off the end of the seat and the footpad rests on the lowest part of the shins.
3. Grab the handles on the machine—or the edges of the seat, if that's more comfortable—and flatten your spine against the backrest.
4. Keeping your back and butt flat against the bench, extend your legs forward until they are straight, knees unlocked. (Do not forcefully swing your legs up, but let your muscles—not momentum—do the work for you.)
5. Pause, lower the weight back down by bending your legs and repeat.

Continue the exercise for a total of 40 seconds, then move on to station #5.

TRICEPS PULLDOWN

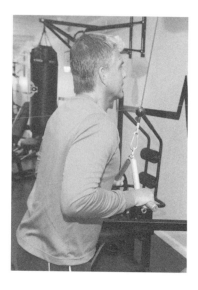
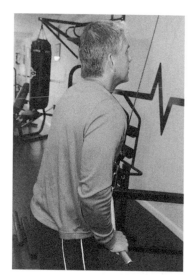

MUSCLES USED: TRICEPS

Here's how to do it:

1. Stand in front of the machine, reach up and grab the bar with both hands. Your grip should be overhand so that your palms are facing down.
2. Tuck your upper arms in to your sides and position your forearms so they are parallel to the floor—your arms should be bent at 90-degree angles.
3. Keeping your back straight and upper arms pinned in to your sides, slowly extend your arms and push the bar down until it reaches the front of your thighs.
4. Squeeze your triceps muscles for a second, then raise the bar back up until your forearms are once again parallel to the floor. Repeat.

Continue the exercise for a total of 40 seconds, then move on to station #6.

Some Cuts facilities use a rope instead of a bar. This works your triceps muscles just as effectively, but you'll have to grab the rope using a different grip than you'll use with a straight bar. Instead of having your palms facing down, grab an end of the rope in each hand and angle your palms slightly in toward each other. Perform the rest of the exercise as you would using a straight bar.

TIP

VERTICAL KNEE RAISE

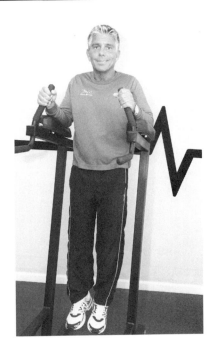 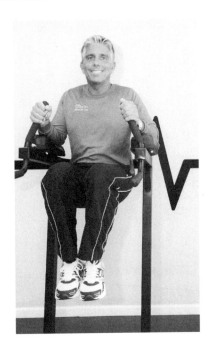

MUSCLES USED: LOWER ABDOMINALS

Here's how to do it:

1. Position yourself in the leg raise machine with your back flat against the pads and your forearms and elbows flat on the pads.
2. Keeping your upper body steady, slowly raise your knees up toward your chest as high as possible. (Don't arch your back; it should stay slightly rounded during the lift.)
3. Slowly lower your legs back down and repeat.

Continue the exercise for a total of 40 seconds, then move on to station #7.

SPIN BIKE

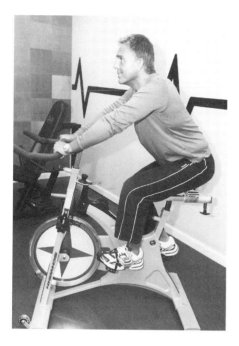

MUSCLES USED: LEGS

Here's how to do it:

1. Sit on the bike seat and slip your feet through the pedal straps.
2. Lean forward over the handle rails, keeping your head slightly up, and begin pedaling.

   Continue the exercise for a total of 40 seconds, then move on to station #8.

Remember to use the brake before getting off the spin bike.

TIP

LEG PRESS

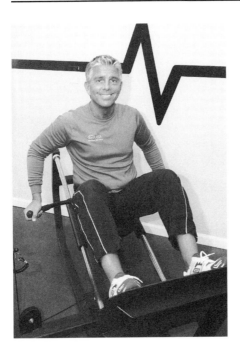

MUSCLES USED: QUADRICEPS, HAMSTRINGS AND GLUTES

Here's how to do it:

1. Sit on the leg press machine and place your feet flat against the crosspiece in front of you—your feet should be around shoulder width apart.

2. Grab the handle grips at your sides for support.

3. Now bend your knees and lower the weight down until your legs are bent at around 90 degrees. (Don't go any farther or your hips will curl up off the seat.)

4. Slowly push the weight back up—using your heels, not your toes—until your legs are straight once again (knees unlocked), then repeat.

Continue the exercise for a total of 40 seconds, then move on to station #9.

BREEZE BIKE

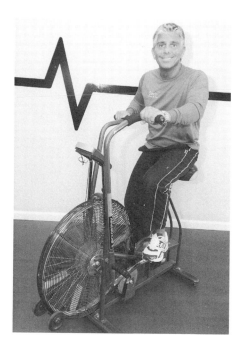

MUSCLES USED: LEGS

Here's how to do it:

1. Sit on the bike seat and grab the handles.
2. Slowly start peddling and moving your arms at the same time.

   Continue the exercise for a total of 40 seconds, then move on to station #10.

Be sure to stop the pedals and arms prior to getting off the bike.

SEATED ABDOMINAL CRUNCH

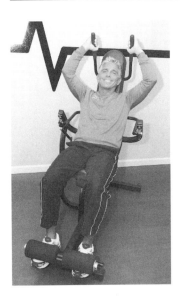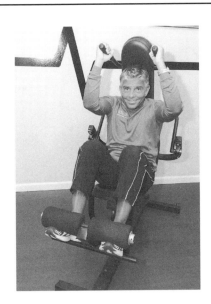

MUSCLES USED: UPPER ABDOMINALS

Here's how to do it:

1. Sit on the seat and place both feet on the bottom bar.
2. Reach overhead behind you and grab the handles with both hands.
3. Maintaining this position, bend at the waist and slowly lower your upper body forward and down—you should feel your abdominal muscles contracting as you go.
4. Slowly raise your torso back up until you are back in the starting position and repeat.

Continue the exercise for a total of 40 seconds, then move on to station #11.

TIP Your feet should stay on the bar at all times, but don't use them to help you pull and push yourself forward and backward. The only muscles you should feel working are your abdominals.

LAT PULLDOWN

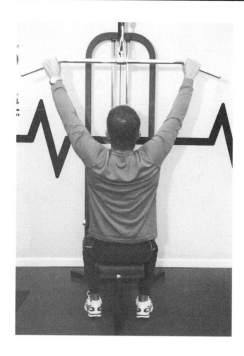 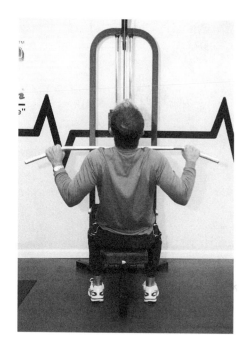

MUSCLES USED: LATISSIMUS DORSI, MIDDLE BACK AND BICEPS

Here's how to do it:

1. Sit down at the machine and tuck your legs snugly underneath the kneepads. Your feet should be flat on the floor.
2. Reach up and grab the bar with an overhand grip—palms facing toward the machine—keeping your hands wider than shoulder width apart.
3. Keeping your legs tucked underneath the pads and your elbows below the bar, slowly pull the bar down until it reaches the top of your chest. Arching your back slightly during the motion is fine, but don't overarch it.
4. Pause, slowly raise the bar back up into the starting position and repeat.

Continue the exercise for a total of 40 seconds, then move on to station #12.

HYDRAULIC STEPPER

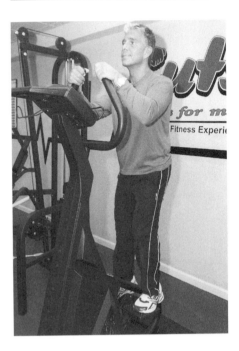

MUSCLES USED: LEGS

Here's how to do it:

1. Step up on to the machine and place your feet flat on the foot pedals.
2. Grab the handles at your sides for support, then begin stepping. The action should feel as though you are walking up a flight of steps.

Continue the exercise for a total of 40 seconds, then move on to station #13.

CABLE CURL

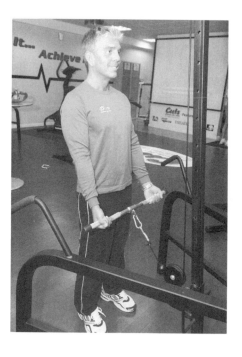 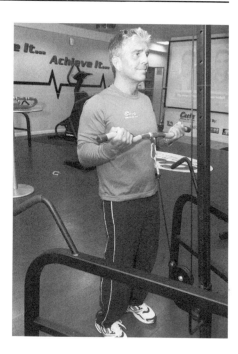

MUSCLES USED: BICEPS

Here's how to do it:

1. Stand facing the low pulley and grab the bar attached to the low cable with an underhand grip—your palms should be facing up.
2. Stand back from the pulley about 1 or 2 feet. (Your arms should be extended straight down in front of you.)
3. Keeping your upper arms pinned to your sides, curl the bar up in a semicircular motion until your hands reach your shoulders. Curl the bar back down to the starting position and repeat.

   Continue the exercise for a total of 40 seconds, then move on to station #14.

SHOULDER PRESS

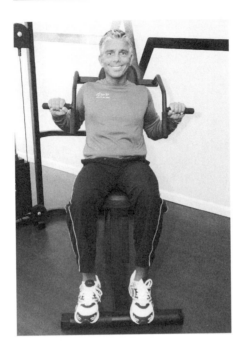 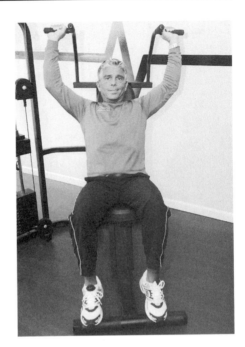

MUSCLES USED: SHOULDERS AND TRICEPS

Here's how to do it:

1. Sit down in the machine and grab the handles with an overhand grip—your palms should be facing forward.
2. Keeping your back flat against the pad, press the handles upward until your arms are straight above your head, elbows unlocked.
3. Lower the handles back down until your hands are directly in front of your shoulders and repeat.

Continue the exercise for a total of 40 seconds, then move on to station #15.

AB SLANT DECLINE BENCH

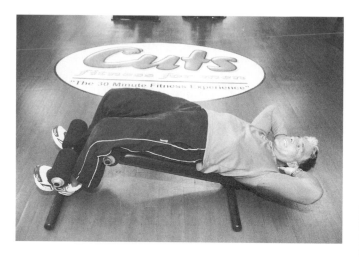

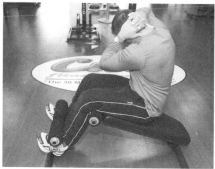

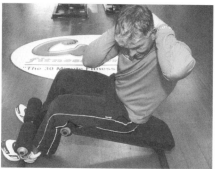

MUSCLES USED: ABDOMINALS AND OBLIQUES

Here's how to do it:

1. Sit down on the decline bench and tuck your feet underneath the pads—this will keep you from sliding as you perform the exercise.

2. Lie flat on the bench and lightly place a hand behind each ear; your elbows should point forward.

3. Keeping your hands in place, slowly curl your torso up and forward as you simultaneously twist to the left—imagine you're trying to touch your right elbow to your left knee.

4. Curl back down, then repeat the exercise, this time curling your torso up and forward as you simultaneously twist to the right—imagine you're trying to touch your left elbow to your right knee.

5. Continue alternating between twisting to the left and right for the remainder of the exercise.

   Continue the exercise for a total of 40 seconds, then move on to station #16.

ROWING MACHINE

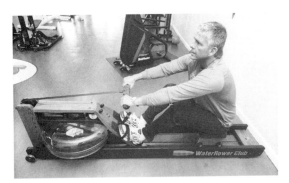 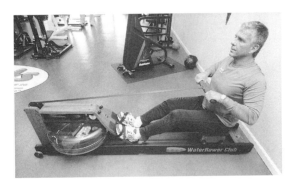

MUSCLES USED: MIDDLE AND LOWER BACK, BICEPS

Here's how to do it:

1. Sit down on the seat with your legs bent, and place your feet shoulder width apart on the platform in front of you.

2. Grab the bar with an overhand grip—your arms should be extended straight out in front of you, hands slightly less than shoulder width apart, with your palms facing down.

3. With your head up and your eyes focused straight in front of you, pull the bar back toward your lower chest as you simultaneously straighten your legs, keeping your elbows close to your sides as you go.

4. Once the bar touches your chest, slowly extend your arms in front of you as you bend your legs and lean your torso slightly forward.

5. Repeat this rowing motion for the duration of the exercise.

   Continue the exercise for a total of 40 seconds, then pause to take your pulse before starting the cycle over by returning to station #1. Your pulse should be within your target heart rate zone. Start back at station #1 and repeat the 16-station circuit twice more for a total of three times.

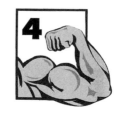

AT HOME

THE CUTS FITNESS FOR MEN HOME WORKOUT

Here's a fact. The three top reasons men say they don't exercise: (1) they can't find the time, (2) they feel intimidated by some "bodybuilding hard-core" gyms, while emasculated by "female-only" health clubs, and (3) they don't want to invest too much money in case they don't keep exercising.

That's where Cuts Fitness For Men has finally redefined how men look at fitness. Every single one of our guy-friendly facilities is easy on the wallet and designed for the guy that wants to get in shape in no time flat, yet doesn't want to be judged for what he can and cannot do. But if you don't have a Cuts Fitness For Men facility in your neighborhood as of yet, you can still experience the same results our members do—right in your very own home.

The Body Cuts home workout achieves the same fitness objectives as the version available in all of our facilities worldwide. All that's required are a few basic pieces of fitness equipment that you can purchase at any sporting goods store—if you don't already have them lying around in your basement:

"Cuts Fitness gave me workout willpower I never had."

LARRY MCCLEAF   AGE: 27 Hanover, PA

"I've always had a problem lacking the willpower to motivate myself to work out at a constant pace or a set time. But because the Body Cuts program forces you to only spend 40 seconds doing each exercise, I never have that problem anymore. I've lost almost 30 pounds since using the workout, and now, I'm not only motivated to exercise, but I find that I can now do a variety of activities without feeling short of breath anymore. Thank you Cuts!"

- A pair of adjustable dumbbells, or ideally, a few pairs of fixed-weight dumbbells, one pair of 10–15 lb. weights, one pair of 20–25 lb. weights and one pair of 30–35 lb. weights (This makes it easier to pick a weight that's best for each exercise, since you may be stronger with some exercises and not as strong with others.)
- A weight bench (A flat bench is fine; none of the moves in the 16-exercise Body Cuts at Home program require you to sit on an incline, which requires a special—more expensive—incline bench.)
- A staircase or a single step

All of this equipment should only run you approximately $100 to $125, which is incredibly inexpensive compared to a traditional gym membership. You can check out www.cutsfitness.com or visit your local sporting goods store. Otherwise, if you look in your local paper, you'll probably find five to six people looking to sell their used dumbbells and weight bench for a lot less. However, if this is still too much for you to invest in just yet, don't worry. In the next chapter, I'll be showing you how to take the official Body Cuts program on the road using minimal equipment—perfect for sticking to the Body Cuts program on vacation, on business, and for those that want to ease their way into trying the program with the least amount of investment.

The Body Cuts home workout is performed in the same exact way as the club version: three times a week, with one day of rest in between each workout. Perform each exercise in the order shown for one set only, using a weight that's heavy enough to let you exhaust your muscles within thirty-five to forty seconds. After you finish all sixteen exercises, you'll take your pulse to make sure your heart rate is in your target heart rate zone.

"Cuts Fitness made me a believer in exercise."

ALBERTO RIVERA AGE: 37 Clifton, NJ

"I never believed in gyms or health clubs, but after joining Cuts Fitness and using the 30-minute Body Cuts program, I realized there was hope. The program has given me the energy that I once had when I was in high school. Thanks, Cuts Fitness, for proving me wrong."

Again, as with the original Body Cuts workout, if your pulse is lower than your target heart rate, you'll increase the amount of weight you're using with each exercise or exercise at a faster pace to up the intensity; if it's higher than your target heart rate, rest until it falls back down in your zone, then try exercising at a lower intensity when you repeat the cycle. Repeat the entire sixteen-exercise circuit for a total of three times.

However, it's important to make sure you are always aware of how much weight you're using. As you get stronger using the program, your muscles will need more resistance to feel as challenged as they did when you first started this program. If you feel that the weight is too light in a particular exercise and that you could easily go longer (for a minute, for example), you need to raise the weight by two-and-a-half to five pounds in that exercise.

did you know that . . .
Just one workout can boost the levels of dopamine, serotonin and norepinephrine—three natural antidepressants that your brain releases into your body? Research at Duke University discovered that subjects who exercised regularly were able to feel less depressed than subjects taking certain antidepression medications.

Before exercising, warm up your muscles
with 3–5 minutes of a low-intensity
cardiovascular exercise, either by jumping in place
or briskly walking around your room.

THE BODY CUTS™
HOME WORKOUT

	Exercise	How to Do It
1	Dumbbell Press	Perform for 40 seconds; move on to exercise #2.
2	Toe Taps	Perform for 40 seconds; move on to exercise #3.
3	Dumbbell Fly	Perform for 40 seconds; move on to exercise #4.
4	Dumbbell Lunge	Perform for 40 seconds; move on to exercise #5.
5	Dumbbell Triceps Extension	Perform for 40 seconds; move on to exercise #6.
6	Reverse Crunch	Perform for 40 seconds; move on to exercise #7.
7	Sliding Squats	Perform for 40 seconds; move on to exercise #8.
8	Dumbbell Squats	Perform for 40 seconds; move on to exercise #9.
9	Toe Taps	Perform for 40 seconds; move on to exercise #10.
10	Traditional Crunch	Perform for 40 seconds; move on to exercise #11.
11	One-Arm Row	Perform for 40 seconds; move on to exercise #12.
12	Sliding Squats	Perform for 40 seconds; move on to exercise #13.
13	Seated Dumbbell Curl	Perform for 40 seconds; move on to exercise #14.
14	Curl Press	Perform for 40 seconds; move on to exercise #15.
15	Double Crunch	Perform for 40 seconds; move on to exercise #16.
16	Dumbbell Row	Perform for 40 seconds; start the cycle over again by starting again with exercise #1. Repeat the cycle 3 times total.

DUMBBELL PRESS

TAKES THE PLACE OF: CHEST PRESS

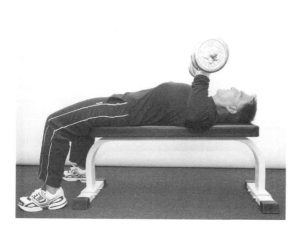 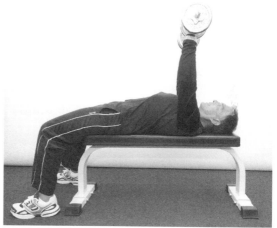

MUSCLES USED: CHEST, SHOULDERS AND TRICEPS

Here's how to do it:

1. Lie on a bench with your feet flat on the floor.
2. Next, grab a weight in each hand and position the weights along the sides of your chest. (Your elbows should be pointing toward the floor.)
3. Now push the weights upward until your arms are fully extended above your chest, elbows unlocked.
4. Slowly lower the weights back along the sides of your chest and repeat.

Continue the exercise for a total of 40 seconds, then move on to exercise #2.

TOE TAPS

TAKES THE PLACE OF: HYDRAULIC STEPPER

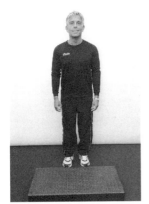 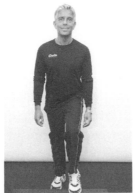 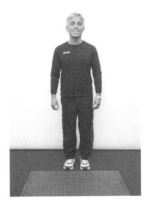 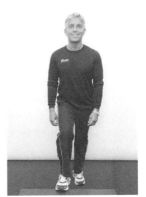

MUSCLES USED: LEGS

Here's how to do it:

1. Stand facing a staircase, feet shoulder width apart, arms by your sides.
2. Hop up onto the step, landing on the toes of your left foot only.
3. Immediately—and carefully—jump off the step, then quickly leap back up, this time landing on the toes of your right foot only.
4. Spring back off the step and continue to repeat the exercise—alternating between your left foot and your right foot.

Continue the exercise for a total of 40 seconds, then move on to exercise #3.

DUMBBELL FLY

TAKES THE PLACE OF: PEC CONTRACTOR

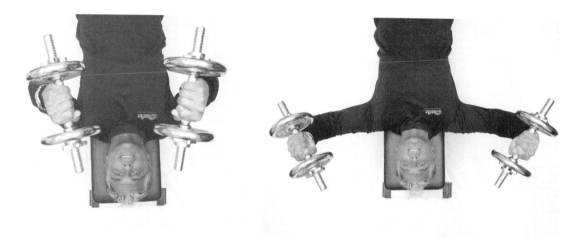

MUSCLES USED: CHEST

Here's how to do it:

1. Lie on a flat bench with knees bent, feet flat on the floor and a dumbbell in each hand.
2. Raise your arms straight up above your chest, elbows slightly bent and palms facing in toward each other.
3. Keeping your arms in this position, slowly sweep your arms down and out to your sides (in an arclike motion) until the weights fall level with your chest.
4. Slowly bring your arms back up in an arclike motion until the weights are once again above your chest, and repeat.

Continue the exercise for a total of 40 seconds, then move on to exercise #4.

DUMBBELL LUNGE

TAKES THE PLACE OF: LEG EXTENSION

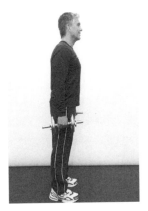 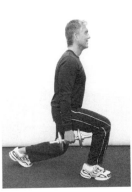 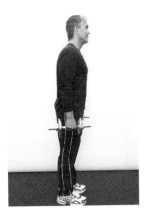 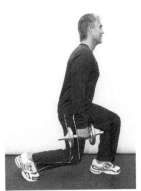

MUSCLES USED: QUADRICEPS

Here's how to do it:

1. Stand straight with your feet shoulder width apart and a dumbbell in each hand, arms down at your sides.
2. Keeping your back straight, take a big step forward with your right foot and gently lean into it until your right thigh is parallel to the floor—your right leg should end up bent at a 90-degree angle. Your left leg should be trailing behind you, with your heel raised off the floor and just the ball of your left foot on the floor.
3. Reverse the motion by pushing off your right foot and stepping back into the starting position, then repeat the lunge, this time stepping forward with your left foot.
4. Repeat the exercise—alternating back and forth between your left and right leg.

Continue the exercise for a total of 40 seconds, then move on to exercise #5.

DUMBBELL TRICEPS EXTENSION

TAKES THE PLACE OF: TRICEPS PULLDOWN

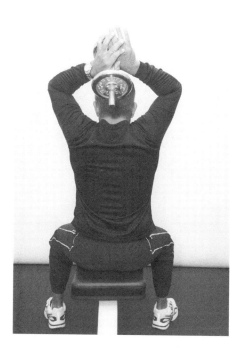 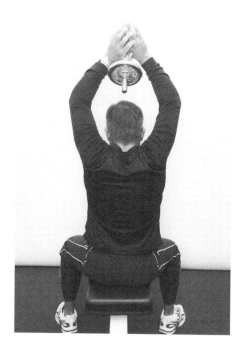

MUSCLES USED: TRICEPS

Here's how to do it:

1. Sit on a chair—or an exercise bench—with your back straight and your feet flat on the floor.
2. Grab a single dumbbell with both hands and raise the weight above your head, rotating it so it's vertical. (The top plate should rest comfortably on the palms of your hands, thumbs around the handle.)
3. Next, slowly lower the weight behind your head until your forearms touch your biceps.
4. Raise the weight back over your head by straightening your arms, and repeat.

   Continue the exercise for a total of 40 seconds, then move on to exercise #6.

REVERSE CRUNCH

TAKES THE PLACE OF: VERTICAL KNEE RAISE

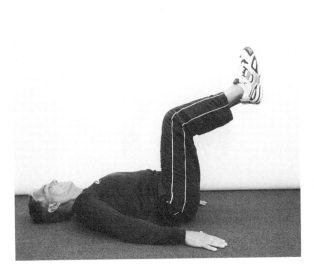
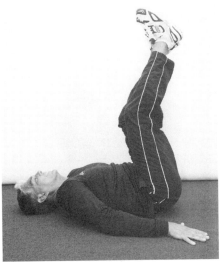

MUSCLES USED: LOWER ABDOMINALS

Here's how to do it:

1. Lie flat on your back with your arms down at your sides, palms flat to the floor.
2. Keeping your legs together, bend your knees and draw them up until your legs form a 90-degree angle. (Your thighs should be perpendicular to the floor.)
3. Next, slowly lift your pelvis off the floor and curl it toward your rib cage. Your knees should automatically curl toward your chest.
4. Pause, then slowly lower your pelvis back down to the floor and repeat.

Continue the exercise for a total of 40 seconds, then move on to exercise #7.

SLIDING SQUATS

TAKES THE PLACE OF: SPIN BIKE

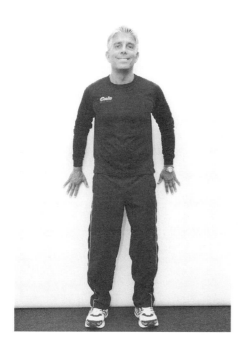 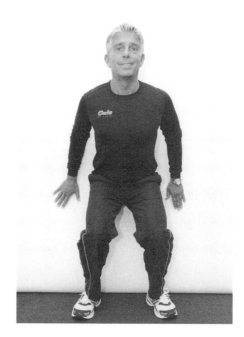

MUSCLES USED: LEGS

Here's how to do it:

1. Stand about 18 inches away from a sturdy wall with your back facing it.
2. Lean back until your entire back is supported by the wall, placing your hands on it for support.
3. Now slowly lower yourself down, sliding down the wall as you go, until your thighs are parallel to the floor.
4. Push yourself back up the wall and repeat.

   Continue the exercise for a total of 40 seconds, then move on to exercise #8.

To make this move harder, try placing your hands on your hips or extending your arms out in front of you.

DUMBBELL SQUATS

TAKES THE PLACE OF: LEG PRESS

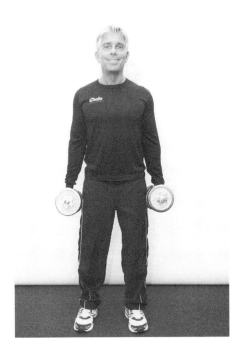 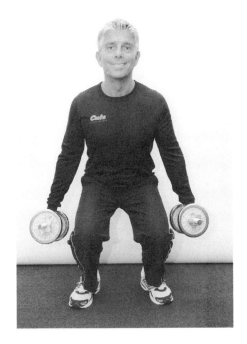

MUSCLES USED: QUADRICEPS, HAMSTRINGS AND GLUTES

Here's how to do it:

1. Stand with a pair of dumbbells in your hands, arms at your sides and feet shoulder width apart.
2. Keeping your back straight and eyes forward, slowly squat down until your thighs are almost perpendicular to the floor.
3. Slowly press yourself back up into a standing position, stopping just short of locking your knees, and repeat.

   Continue the exercise for a total of 40 seconds, then move on to exercise #9.

TIP

If you have a hard time squatting all the way down, try a Quarter Dumbbell Squat instead—you'll still train the same leg muscles. Just squat down about 6 to 8 inches, then rise back up into a standing position.

TOE TAPS

TAKES THE PLACE OF: BREEZE BIKE

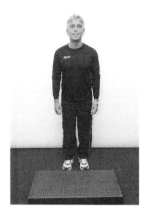 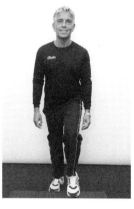 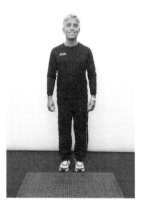 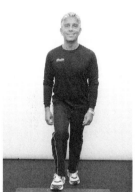

MUSCLES USED: LEGS

Here's how to do it:

1. Stand facing a staircase, feet shoulder width apart, arms by your sides.
2. Hop up onto the step, landing on the toes of your left foot only.
3. Immediately—and carefully—jump off the step, then quickly leap back up, this time landing on the toes of your right foot only.
4. Spring back off the step and continue to repeat the exercise—alternating between your left foot and your right foot.

Continue the exercise for a total of 40 seconds, then move on to exercise #10.

TRADITIONAL CRUNCH

TAKES THE PLACE OF: SEATED ABDOMINAL CRUNCH

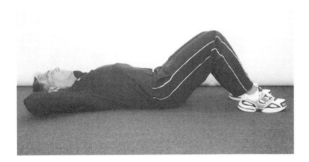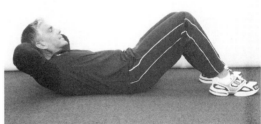

MUSCLES USED: UPPER ABDOMINALS

Here's how to do it:

1. Lie flat on the floor with your knees bent and your feet spread shoulder width apart.
2. Place your hands along the sides of your head so that they're lightly touching your head behind your ears.
3. As you begin to exhale, slowly curl your head and torso toward your knees until your shoulder blades are off the floor, keeping your feet flat and your hands alongside your head. Imagine that you're drawing your ribs to your hips, as if your midsection were an accordion.
4. Pause, lower yourself back down—inhaling as you go—and repeat.

Continue the exercise for a total of 40 seconds, then move on to exercise #11.

ONE-ARM ROW

TAKES THE PLACE OF: LAT PULLDOWN

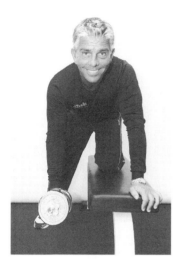 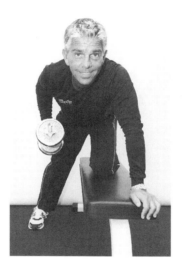 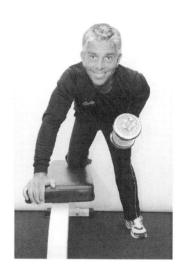

MUSCLES USED: LATISSIMUS DORSI, MIDDLE BACK AND BICEPS

Here's how to do it:

1. Stand with your left side to an exercise bench and a dumbbell in your right hand. (If you don't have a bench, you can use the end of a bed.)
2. Rest your left hand and knee on the bench, bend at the waist and let your right arm hang down toward the floor, palm facing in toward the bench.
3. Slowly draw the weight up close to the body until it reaches your chest.
4. Lower the weight back down until your right arm is straight and repeat.
5. After 4–8 repetitions, place the weight in your left hand, switch positions on the bench by placing your right hand and knee on the bench and repeat the exercise—this time performing the row with your left arm for another 4–8 repetitions.

Continue the exercise for a total of 40 seconds, then move on to exercise #12.

12

SLIDING SQUATS

TAKES THE PLACE OF: HYDRAULIC STEPPER

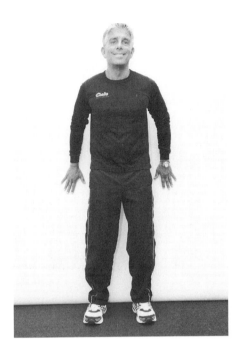 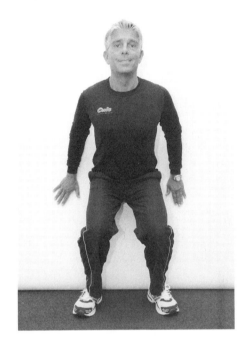

MUSCLES USED: LEGS

Here's how to do it:

1. Stand about 18 inches away from a sturdy wall with your back facing it.

2. Lean back until your entire back is leaning on the wall, placing your hands on it for support.

3. Now slowly lower yourself down, sliding down the wall as you go, until your thighs are parallel to the floor.

4. Push yourself back up the wall and repeat.

Continue the exercise for a total of 40 seconds, then move on to exercise #13.

TIP

To make this move harder, try placing your hands on your hips or extending your arms out in front of you.

SEATED DUMBBELL CURL

TAKES THE PLACE OF: CABLE CURL

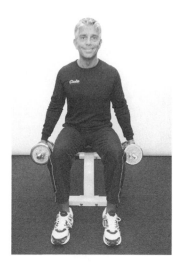 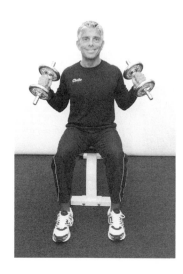 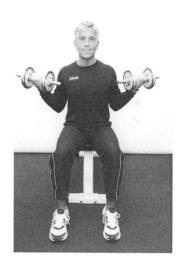

MUSCLES USED: BICEPS

Here's how to do it:

1. Sit on the edge of a chair with a dumbbell in each hand, arms hanging down at your sides, palms facing each other.
2. Keeping your back straight, curl both dumbbells up toward your shoulders. Your elbows should be pointing down toward the floor.
3. Pause, lower the weights back down to your sides and repeat.

   Continue the exercise for a total of 40 seconds, then move on to exercise #14.

CURL PRESS

TAKES THE PLACE OF: SHOULDER PRESS

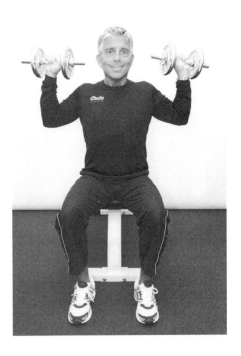 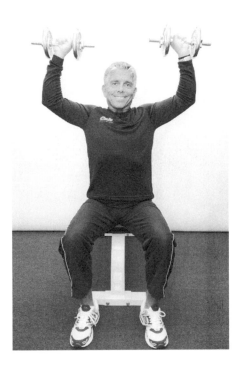

MUSCLES USED: SHOULDERS AND TRICEPS

Here's how to do it:

1. Sit on a chair (or the edge of a weight bench), feet firmly on the floor with a dumbbell in each hand.
2. Bring the weights to the sides of your shoulders, palms facing out.
3. Slowly press the weights over your head, keeping your back straight as you go.
4. Lower them back to your shoulders and repeat.

Continue the exercise for a total of 40 seconds, then move on to exercise #15.

DOUBLE CRUNCH

TAKES THE PLACE OF: AB SLANT DECLINE BENCH

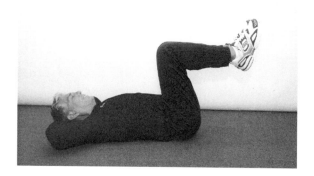
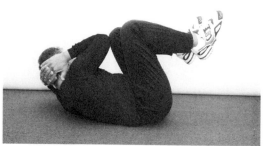

MUSCLES USED: UPPER AND LOWER ABDOMINALS

Here's how to do it:

1. Lie flat with your knees bent, feet flat on the floor.
2. Touch your hands lightly to the sides of your head, pointing your elbows toward your knees. This is the starting position.
3. Now curl your torso up toward your midsection, while simultaneously raising your knees toward your elbows. Your elbows should touch the front of your thighs in the middle—if they don't, that's OK. Just try to point your elbows toward your thighs.
4. Lower yourself back down—your head, shoulders and feet should all be touching the floor—and repeat.

   Continue the exercise for a total of 40 seconds, then move on to exercise #16.

DUMBBELL ROW

TAKES THE PLACE OF: ROWING MACHINE

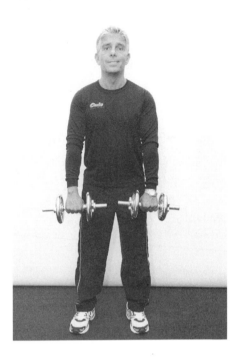 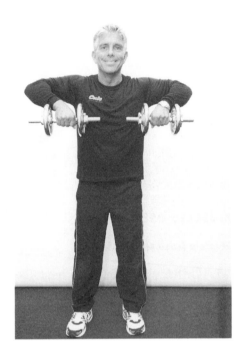

MUSCLES USED: UPPER BACK AND SHOULDERS

Here's how to do it:

1. Stand straight with a light dumbbell in each hand and your arms hanging straight down in front of you—your hands should be turned so that your palms are facing your thighs.
2. Keeping your back straight, slowly raise the weights straight up and close to your body until the dumbbells come up just below your chin.
3. Pause, lower the weights back down in front of you until your arms are straight and repeat.

   Continue the exercise for a total of 40 seconds, then pause to take your pulse before starting the cycle over by returning to exercise #1. Your pulse should be within your target zone. Start back at exercise #1 and repeat the 16-exercise cycle twice more for a total of three times.

Tune Up Your Day
to See More Results

FOLLOWING THE Body Cuts workout may be the secret to a healthier new you, but there are a few additional things you can do that can help you reap more benefits from the plan. Here are three tricks to try on a regular basis to make sure you get every single benefit your body deserves:

Check your pulse regularly

Pushing yourself too hard in exercise can prevent your body from having enough time to recover. This can lead to something experts call "overtraining," which can stall your results and even increase your risk of getting injured. To prevent it from happening to you, try slowing down for a week, then take your pulse when you wake up in the morning. Then, return to your normal schedule and take your pulse first thing each morning. If it rises faster than seven beats a minute, you're overtraining and should slow the pace down a bit.

Discover the best time for your body

Some experts believe that your body has several peak energy cycles throughout the day. That means you may be trying to exercise when you're mentally and physically at your worst. If possible, try to exercise at different times of the day to find when your energy level is at its highest.

Be aware of your extracurricular activities

Staying active is what the Cuts Fitness program is all about, but getting involved in a sport or participating in any activity that's physically demanding could keep your body from getting the rest it needs to help your muscles grow. I want you to stay active, but try to figure out which muscles you're using when you're active, then try to take it easy on those muscles when using any of the Body Cuts workouts. If you're not sure which muscles are being used, listen to your body the morning after you play a sport and see which muscles are sore.

ON THE ROAD

THE CUTS FITNESS FOR MEN
NO-EXCUSES WORKOUT

I'll never forget the first client that came up to me disappointed about the Body Cuts program.

He wasn't disappointed with the results, mind you. He had seen instant results, within just a few short weeks, and wanted to keep those results coming. The problem was that he had joined Cuts Fitness For Men when things at work were slow, but when his busy season started up again, he knew he'd be on the road for weeks on end, with no guarantee he would find a Cuts facility in whatever town he blew into each night.

I knew that feeling of dread, because I lived it myself. That moment of getting your exercise back on track for a few days, only to have a huge workload interfere with your workouts. One step forward, three steps back—that's how it always felt back then. But this time, I knew that if my mission was to get men back into exercise at any age, then there couldn't be any barriers. There couldn't be any excuses—whether it's traveling for work, or vacation or just having limited funds that's preventing someone from sticking with the program. Like I said, the whole idea of combining many of the exercises in the Body Cuts workout was born out of necessity.

"I never have to wait to work out."

ERIC HORMEL AGE: 35 Hanover, PA

"The biggest problem for me was getting a worthwhile workout during the only time I had to exercise—my lunch hour. Oftentimes, I would spend an hour in the gym exercising, but half of that time was waiting around on other people just to use a machine. The Body Cuts program is so structured that it takes the drudgery out of exercise. Now I'm 27 pounds lighter, I've dropped my body fat down to 14.3 percent, I have more energy to play golf, but most importantly, I have the satisfaction of feeling better about myself."

And so was the Body Cuts No-Excuses workout.

Taking all of the principles and goals into account—and looking at the sixteen exercises that make up the original Body Cuts workout, I found a way to re-create the same strength-training and cardiovascular benefits using minimal equipment. All you'll be using for this sixteen-station circuit is a sturdy chair, a step (or a sturdy box that can support your weight) and a pair of resistance cords—which are basically cords made from surgical tubing or rubber that work your muscles as you push, pull or curl them and, best of all, they are cheap (around $15) and take up no space at all—just roll them up and go—so you can bring them anywhere.

A stretch cord, you say? Isn't that something that women use? If that was your first impression, that's where you're wrong. If you're like most men, you probably assume that strength training means working out with dumbbells, barbells and other weight-assisted machines. The truth is, strength training is any form of "resistance training," which means any type of exercise where your muscles have to exert force against some form of resistance. That resistance can come from anything: weights, cables, stretch cords, even your own body weight.

"When my husband joined Cuts Fitness For Men, he made a commitment to exercising and leading a healthy lifestyle, and has lost 35 pounds in the process. I'm proud that he has followed through as this has not only made him more fit and healthy, but has had the same effect for our entire family. We now eat better and even try to walk together as well. Thanks, Cuts!"

—Carol-Ann Manfria on her husband, DON

Mind you, certain types of resistance can be easier on your joints, tendons and ligaments than others, but for the most part, your muscles really can't tell whether the resistance they're working against is metal, rubber or your own body. All they know is that they're being worked—and challenged—on a regular basis, which forces them to get stronger and look better over time.

The Body Cuts No-Excuses workout is a full-body workout that will give your body everything it needs to stay fit, using a combination of body-weight exercises along with a few movements that require you to either step on a resistance cord or tie it to a sturdy object so you can pull and stretch it to train your muscles. It's also performed in the same exact way as the club version: three times a week, with one day of rest in between each workout. Perform each exercise in the order shown for one set only.

Because many of the exercises in the program use your body weight as resistance (such as push-ups, chair squats, etc.), you may have difficulty doing certain exercises for a full forty seconds if you're heavier. That's fine; just try to do as many repetitions of these exercises as you can and rest for the remainder of the forty seconds. (If you're afraid that taking these little breaks will negate some of the benefits of the program, don't worry. Remember, doing less because you weigh more also means you're making your muscles lift much more weight than the average guy, so you're challenging your muscles regardless.)

As for any of the exercises that require a stretch cord, be sure to adjust the cord during each exercise so that it exhausts the muscles you're trying to work within thirty-five to forty seconds. If the exercise feels too easy, just stand farther away from where you've attached the cord, or if you're standing on the center of the cord, try grabbing the cords farther down from each end. These tweaks help make the stretch cord tighter before you start the exercise, which makes it harder to use it when you perform the move.

After you finish all sixteen exercises, you'll take your pulse to make sure your heart rate is in your target heart rate zone. Again, as with the original Body Cuts program, if your pulse is lower than your target heart rate, try adjusting the cords to make them tighter before you start the exercise, or just exercise at a faster pace to up the intensity; if your pulse is higher than your target heart rate, rest until it falls back down in your zone, then try exercising at a lower intensity when you repeat the cycle. Repeat the entire sixteen-exercise circuit for a total of three times.

Before exercising, warm up your muscles with 3–5 minutes of a low-intensity cardiovascular exercise, either by jumping in place or briskly walking around your room.

THE BODY CUTS™
NO-EXCUSES WORKOUT

	Exercise	How to Do It
1	Push-ups	Perform for 40 seconds; move on to exercise #2.
2	Jog/Walk in Place	Perform for 40 seconds; move on to exercise #3.
3	Plank	Perform for 40 seconds; move on to exercise #4.
4	Step Lunges	Perform for 40 seconds; move on to exercise #5.
5	Chair Dip	Perform for 40 seconds; move on to exercise #6.
6	Seated Crisscrosses	Perform for 40 seconds; move on to exercise #7.
7	Bridge	Perform for 40 seconds; move on to exercise #8.
8	Chair Squats	Perform for 40 seconds; move on to exercise #9.
9	Simulated Jump Rope	Perform for 40 seconds; move on to exercise #10.
10	Reaching Crunch	Perform for 40 seconds; move on to exercise #11.
11	Resistance Band Row	Perform for 40 seconds; move on to exercise #12.
12	Jog/Walk in Place	Perform for 40 seconds; move on to exercise #13.
13	Resistance Band Biceps Curl	Perform for 40 seconds; move on to exercise #14.
14	Resistance Band Lateral Raise	Perform for 40 seconds; move on to exercise #15.
15	Twist Crunch	Perform for 40 seconds; move on to exercise #16.
16	Hyperextensions	Perform for 40 seconds; start the cycle over again by starting again with exercise #1. Repeat the cycle 3 times total.

PUSH-UPS

TAKES THE PLACE OF: CHEST PRESS

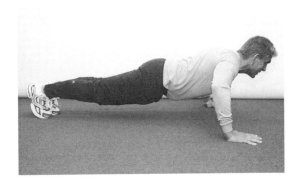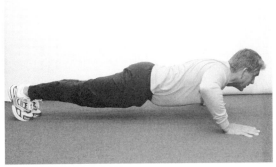

MUSCLES USED: CHEST, SHOULDERS AND TRICEPS

Here's how to do it:

1. Place your hands flat on the floor (shoulder width apart) with your arms straight and elbows unlocked.
2. Straighten your legs behind you, drawing your feet together.
3. Rise up on your toes so the top of the balls of your feet are touching the floor. Your body should be one straight line from your feet to your head, your eyes focused straight down at the ground below.
4. Without moving your head, slowly lower yourself until your upper arms are parallel to the ground.
5. Pause, slowly push yourself back up, and repeat.

Continue the exercise for a total of 40 seconds, then move on to exercise #2.

TIP Can't do a full push-up just yet? Don't worry, you will in time. But until then, try doing them on your knees to start. A normal push-up angles your body so that you're pressing about 60 percent of your body weight. That can mean a lot if you're currently overweight. However, resting on your knees instead of your feet changes the angle of the movement, so you press around 35 to 40 percent of your body weight instead.

JOG/WALK IN PLACE

TAKES THE PLACE OF: HYDRAULIC STEPPER

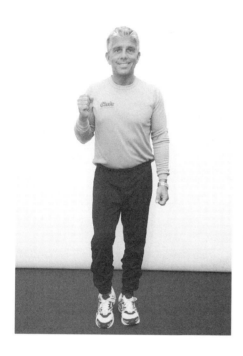 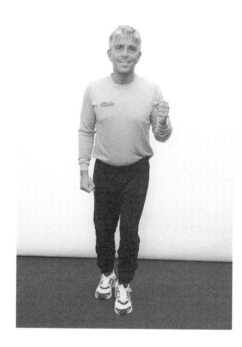

MUSCLES USED: LEGS

Here's how to do it:

1. Stand straight with your arms at your sides, elbows bent at 90 degrees.
2. Walk briskly—or jog—in place, pumping your arms backward and forward as you go.

Continue the exercise for a total of 40 seconds, then move on to exercise #3.

PLANK

TAKES THE PLACE OF: PEC CONTRACTOR

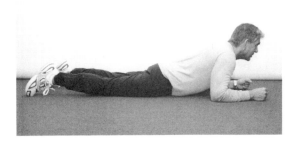 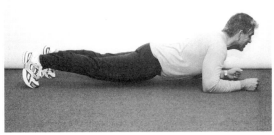

MUSCLES USED: CHEST, SHOULDERS AND ABS

Here's how to do it:

1. Lie flat on your stomach with your legs straight and your arms bent at your sides—your elbows should be pointing back toward your feet; your fists positioned by your shoulders, palms facing in.
2. Push yourself up off the floor so that you're resting only on your forearms and your toes. Your arms should end up bent at 90-degree angles.
3. Keeping your abs held in and your head down—your body should form a straight line from your head to your feet—hold this position for as long as possible, or for the allotted time.

Continue the exercise for a total of 40 seconds, then move on to exercise #4.

STEP LUNGES

TAKES THE PLACE OF: LEG EXTENSION

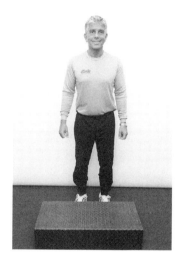 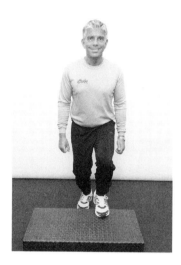 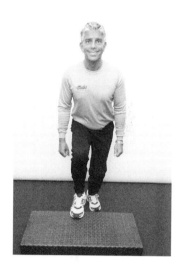

MUSCLES USED: QUADRICEPS

Here's how to do it:

1. Stand about three feet in front of a staircase. Let your arms hang at your sides, palms facing in toward your legs, with your feet about six inches apart.
2. Keeping your back straight, step forward with your left foot and place it directly on the first step.
3. Keep leaning forward until your left thigh is almost parallel to the floor, then gently push yourself back into the starting position.
4. Repeat the same move with the right leg. Continue to alternate between stepping forward with your left foot and your right foot.

Continue the exercise for a total of 40 seconds, then move on to exercise #5.

CHAIR DIP

TAKES THE PLACE OF: TRICEPS PULLDOWN

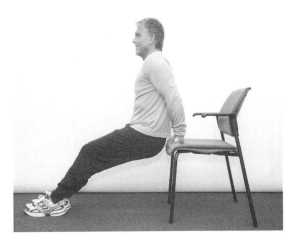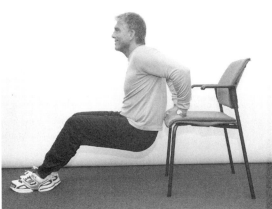

MUSCLES USED: TRICEPS

Here's how to do it:

1. Place your hands on the back of a sturdy chair, positioning them so that your fingers are pointing in toward your lower back.
2. Keeping your hands in place, slowly step forward until your legs are in front of you. Your arms should be straight, elbows unlocked, supporting your weight behind you.
3. Next, slowly lower yourself as far as you can and bring your butt as close to the floor as possible.
4. Press yourself back up until your arms are straight, elbows unlocked, and repeat.

Continue the exercise for a total of 40 seconds, then move on to exercise #6.

SEATED CRISSCROSSES

TAKES THE PLACE OF: VERTICAL KNEE RAISE

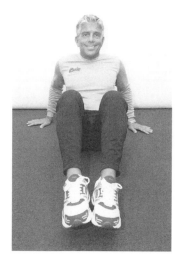 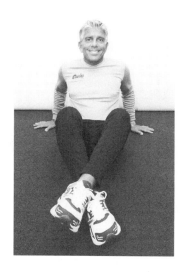 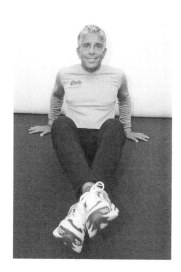

MUSCLES USED: LOWER ABDOMINALS

Here's how to do it:

1. Sit on the floor with your legs in front of you, knees bent at 90-degree angles.
2. Reach back and comfortably place your hands flat on the floor behind you to support yourself.
3. Keeping your legs bent, raise your feet a few inches off the ground. This is the starting position.
4. Keeping your feet suspended just above the floor, cross your left foot above your right without letting them touch.
5. Pause, uncross your feet and repeat, this time placing your right foot above your left.
6. Keep alternating back and forth at a brisk pace.

   Continue the exercise for a total of 40 seconds, then move on to exercise #7.

BRIDGE

TAKES THE PLACE OF: SPIN BIKE

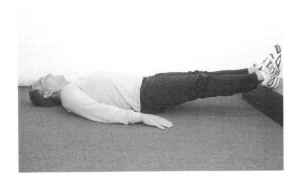 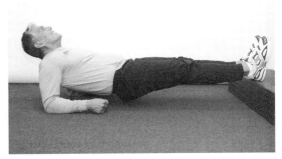

MUSCLES USED: HAMSTRINGS AND GLUTES

Here's how to do it:

1. Lie on your back on a mat (or carpeted floor) with your knees bent and your heels resting on the edge of a step. (If you don't have a step, resting your heels on the edge of your couch will do.)
2. Relax your arms by your sides.
3. Contract your abs, then press down through your heels to lift your pelvis, waist, then upper back off the floor. Really squeeze your abs throughout the exercise to avoid overarching your back.
4. Pause, return to the starting position by lowering yourself back down to the floor, and repeat.

Continue the exercise for a total of 40 seconds, then move on to exercise #8.

CHAIR SQUATS

TAKES THE PLACE OF: LEG PRESS

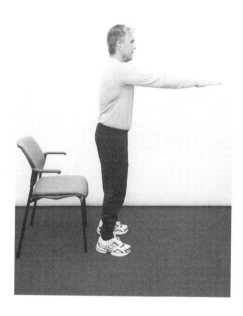 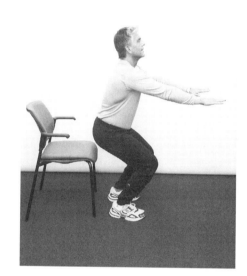

MUSCLES USED: QUADRICEPS, HAMSTRINGS AND GLUTES

Here's how to do it:

1. Stand with your back facing away from a sturdy chair, your feet shoulder width apart and your arms extended in front of you.
2. Keeping your head and back straight, slowly squat down until your butt touches the chair.
3. Push yourself back up into a standing position and repeat.

   Continue the exercise for a total of 40 seconds, then move on to exercise #9.

SIMULATED JUMP ROPE

TAKES THE PLACE OF: BREEZE BIKE

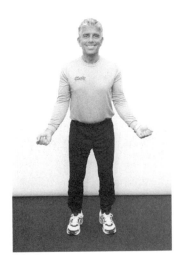
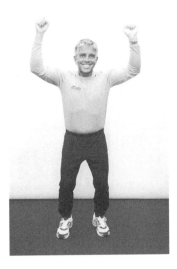
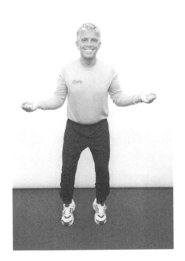

MUSCLES USED: LEGS

Here's how to do it:

(For this exercise, you don't need a jump rope. You'll just be mimicking the motions instead—it burns the same amount of calories without requiring as much coordination or the space to use a rope.)

1. Stand as if you were holding a jump rope—your legs should be straight with your feet together (knees unlocked) and your arms down by your sides.
2. Turn your arms as if you were swinging the rope overhead.
3. As the "rope" reaches your feet, jump up with both feet—just hopping an inch or so off the floor will do—to let the rope pass under.
4. Keep skipping rope at a pace that's challenging for you.

Continue the exercise for a total of 40 seconds, then move on to exercise #10.

REACHING CRUNCH

TAKES THE PLACE OF: SEATED ABDOMINAL CRUNCH

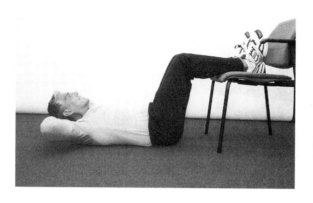 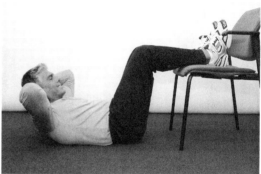

MUSCLES USED: UPPER ABDOMINALS

Here's how to do it:

1. Lie with your arms extended straight behind your head, hands clasped together.
2. Next, raise your feet and place them on a chair so that your legs are bent at a 90-degree angle.
3. Press your heels down into the chair (to keep the hip flexors from indirectly doing all the work) then curl your torso forward until your shoulder blades are off the floor, keeping your arms straight and alongside your head.
4. Pause, lower yourself back down and repeat.

   Continue the exercise for a total of 40 seconds, then move on to exercise #11.

If you feel more comfortable, you can cross your arms over your chest or touch your hands lightly alongside of each ear instead.

TIP

RESISTANCE BAND ROW

TAKES THE PLACE OF: LAT PULLDOWN

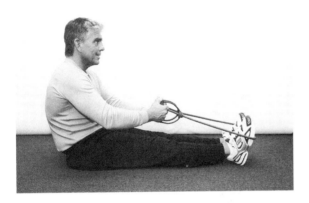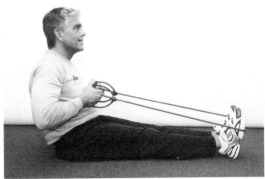

MUSCLES USED: UPPER AND LOWER BACK

Here's how to do it:

1. Sit on the floor with your legs extended straight out in front of you.
2. Loop a piece of tubing over your feet and grab an end in each hand—your arms should be extended in front of you toward your feet. If there is slack in the resistance band, then grab it farther down each end.
3. Keeping your back perpendicular to the floor, squeeze your shoulder blades together, then pull your hands toward you as close to your chest as you can.
4. Pause, slowly extend your arms back out in front of you once more and repeat.

Continue the exercise for a total of 40 seconds, then move on to exercise #12.

JOG/WALK IN PLACE

TAKES THE PLACE OF: HYDRAULIC STEPPER

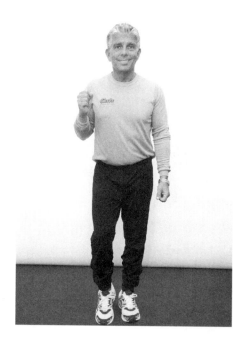 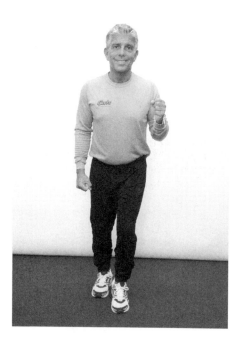

MUSCLES USED: LEGS

Here's how to do it:

1. Stand straight with your arms at your sides, elbows bent at 90 degrees.
2. Walk briskly—or jog—in place, pumping your arms backward and forward as you go.

   Continue the exercise for a total of 40 seconds, then move on to exercise #13.

13

RESISTANCE BAND BICEPS CURL

TAKES THE PLACE OF: CABLE CURL

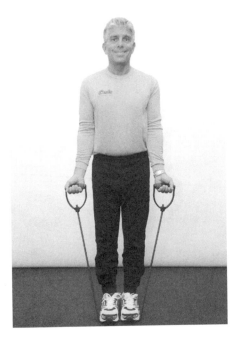
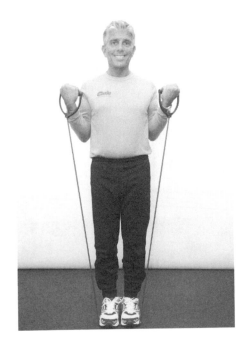

MUSCLES USED: BICEPS

Here's how to do it:

1. Grab a piece of tubing in each hand and step on the middle of the band with both feet.
2. Stand with your arms at your sides and your palms facing forward.
3. Keeping your upper arms tucked against your sides, slowly bend your elbows and curl your fists up until they reach the front of your shoulders.
4. Curl your fists back down until your arms are straight again and repeat.

Continue the exercise for a total of 40 seconds, then move on to exercise #14.

RESISTANCE BAND LATERAL RAISE

TAKES THE PLACE OF: SHOULDER PRESS

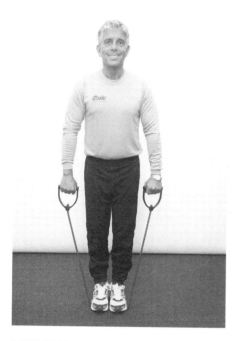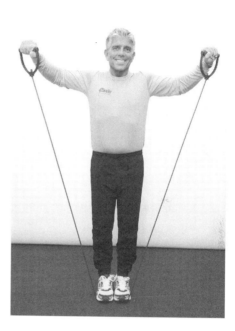

MUSCLES USED: SHOULDERS

Here's how to do it:

1. Grab an end of tubing in each hand and step on the middle of the band with both feet.
2. Stand with your arms at your sides and your palms facing your thighs.
3. Keeping your arms straight, slowly raise them out to your sides until they are parallel to the floor. (You'll look like the letter T.)
4. Lower your arms back down to your sides, then raise them up again, this time straight out in front of your body.
5. Lower your arms back down and continue to alternate between both movements (raising your arms out to the sides, then raising them out in front of you).

Continue the exercise for a total of 40 seconds, then move on to exercise #15.

TWIST CRUNCH

TAKES THE PLACE OF: AB SLANT DECLINE BENCH

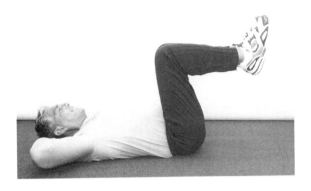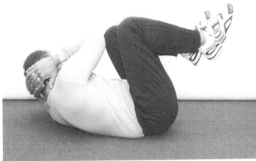

MUSCLES USED: ABDOMINALS AND OBLIQUES

Here's how to do it:

1. Lie flat on your back with your legs bent at a 90-degree angle.
2. Lift your legs up until your thighs are perpendicular to the floor.
3. Touch your hands lightly to the sides of your head with your elbows pointing toward your legs.
4. To start, slowly lift your shoulders off the ground and twist your body to the left so your right elbow reaches out toward your thighs. At the same time, draw *both* knees in to meet your elbow.
5. Lower yourself back down and repeat the movement, this time twisting to the right so that your left elbow meets your knees.
6. Continue to repeat the exercise, alternating between twisting from the left and twisting from the right.

Continue the exercise for a total of 40 seconds, then move on to exercise #16.

HYPEREXTENSIONS

TAKES THE PLACE OF: ROWING MACHINE

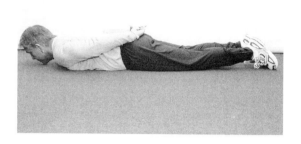 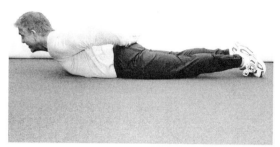

MUSCLES USED: LOWER BACK

Here's how to do it:

1. Lie facedown on your stomach with your arms behind you and your fingers interlaced behind your lower back.
2. Raise your arms up behind you, pressing your knuckles toward your feet, then slowly raise your chest off the floor as high as you comfortably can—your feet and legs should stay on the floor.
3. Pause at the top, lower your chest and head back down to the floor and repeat.

Continue the exercise for a total of 40 seconds, then pause to take your pulse before starting the cycle over by returning to exercise #1. Your pulse should be within your target zone. Start back at exercise #1 and repeat the 16-exercise cycle twice more for a total of three times.

Instant Exercise Motivation!

EXERCISING ON A consistent basis, no matter how energizing the workout, can sometimes feel less inspiring. To rekindle your regime, these three simple tricks can make a world of difference to your workouts:

Work out with someone

Try exercising with your significant other. (Cuts Fitness may be for men only, but you can do this at home.) Research from Indiana University at Bloomington found that couples that worked out together exercised more regularly than couples that chose to exercise away from each other—just 6 percent of the couples quit working out after a short period of time, while 43 percent quit when working out solo. If you can't get your partner to do it, anyone will do, so long as they are as serious about exercise as you are.

Wear clothing you like seeing yourself in

If you don't like what you see in the mirror, it can hurt your motivation to do something about it. Some men find that they race through their routines or just quit altogether when they suffer from a lower sense of self-esteem because of how they look. Instead, spend a few bucks on some exercise clothes you feel comfortable in—anything that leaves you feeling slimmer, stronger and more fit will do. Or put your favorite T-shirts, shorts, etc., aside and use them only for exercise. Liking what you're wearing will make you want to wear these clothes more often, which keeps many guys on track by making them want to exercise more often.

Move yourself around as you work out

Creating a sense of newness to your workout when you're using the same routine over and over again can be as simple as altering your view. If you always exercise in the same room in your house, try a different room for a change—or just angle your chair, bench or body so you're facing another direction. Enjoying a new view, even if it's only a slight difference, can change your exercise experience so it feels fresh again.

THREE

TAKING YOUR WORKOUT TO THE NEXT LEVEL

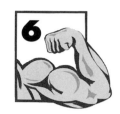

"CUT" OUT THE BAD FOODS

ARE YOU READY FOR THE BIGGEST REASON OF ALL TO LOSE WEIGHT?

Research has shown that dropping just 5 percent of your total body fat can have a profound effect on reducing your chances of many cardiovascular and arterial complications, as well as a variety of weight-induced diseases. That means if you're two hundred pounds right now, losing just ten pounds of body fat can make *that* much of an impact on your life right now.

That's why I want you to lose the extra weight you've been carrying around all this time. As I said before, it's not just about better looks, it's about a better life. The Body Cuts program will go a long way in helping you lose weight fast, and for many of you, it will be all you'll need to slim down. However, I also know that working up a sweat isn't the only way to keep your growing belly in check and those extra pounds at bay.

"22 pounds gone for good . . . and no waiting."

BRENT BUXTON   AGE: 44 Alpharetta, GA

"Before looking into Cuts Fitness For Men, I was in really bad shape with a lower back problem. It was hard for me just to get out of my La-Z-boy because my joints ached so badly. I also had a problem eating well and I never had any type of regular exercise routine in my life.

"When my chiropractor told me exercise would help my lower back, I didn't know what to do. I didn't like conventional gyms because they were always crowded and forced their members to wait in lines for equipment. With the Body Cuts program, I never had to wait in line for a piece of equipment. Best of all, I haven't seen my chiropractor in over 2 years. Thanks Cuts Fitness, for helping me feel as healthy as I did in my 20s."

Why You'll Never Have to Diet Using the Body Cuts™ Program

There are two major mistakes most men make when it comes to weight loss.

The first? Believing you can *always* reach your ideal weight through just exercise alone. The second? Thinking you can *always* achieve the same goal by dieting alone. The truth is, it doesn't matter how much you sweat or starve yourself, the best way to guarantee results always come from the right combination of a solid exercise regime and a sound nutrition plan. The problem is that when it comes to dieting and nutrition, most older men go about it the wrong way, especially when weight loss is their main goal.

Trying to lose fat by restricting what you eat—which so many guys try to do out of desperation—is the route a lot of men take to trim up. The logic is that limiting what you eat leaves your body no choice but to look for stored sources of energy elsewhere, such as all that excess body fat you've been looking to shed. The problem is that when you starve your body by overly limiting the number of calories you eat on a daily basis, it doesn't just burn more body fat for energy.

did you know that . . .
For every one hundred calories you burn during exercise, your body will roughly burn an extra fifteen calories afterward? That's because the Body Cuts program briefly boosts your metabolism, so it continues to stay at an elevated level for several minutes after you're finished exercising.

It also burns any excess muscle tissue.

That means that the muscle you're so desperately trying to hold onto right now could be eaten up—literally—if you're not smart about turning to the right nutritional plan. I'm not talking about starting any of the fad diets you've seen so many other guys try and fail in the past. I'm talking about making a few smart decisions when it comes to what, when and how you eat. It doesn't take that much sacrifice in your diet to make an impact on your health and trim off those last few pounds that may still be hanging on.

The Body Cuts program not only helps you build quality muscle tissue, but strength training also lets your body know to leave your muscles "off the menu" when your body is burning the fat. If you typically eat fewer calories than the average man consumes or just consider yourself a calorie-conscious exerciser, that means you won't lose a single ounce of muscle from all the hard work you've invested using the Body Cuts program to firm up and reshape your body.

And, unlike many strength-training programs that only work your muscles, the Body Cuts program also elevates your heart simultaneously, so you'll use more stored fat and calories for energy. That's why our Cuts Fitness For Men members find themselves spending less time being meticulous with their nutritional plan throughout the week. The fat-burning, muscle-sparing benefits of the Body Cuts program make it easier to add just a few subtle changes to your eating habits, so you never have to see another—or use another—diet ever again.

"I've lost 47 pounds and counting."

DAVID VEGA AGE: 24 Hesperia, CA

"Lack of self-motivation was my biggest problem. I would work out for a week, then quit for two months. The end result left me weighing in at 193 unhealthy pounds. For health reasons, I turned to Cuts Fitness and the results came quick. Now, exercising just three times a week for 30 minutes a session, I have more energy and have dropped from 193 pounds to 146 pounds. I can't believe it was that simple to reshape my body."

Commonsense Eating: The Cuts Way

To lose those last stubborn pounds, you don't need to diet, you just need to follow a few simple dos and don'ts to help in your battle of the bulge. Here are the easiest nutritional tips that can make the biggest difference in a man's life, with the least amount of effort:

DO . . . CUT your meals in half. Most men tend to eat two to three large meals a day, but try chopping your meals in half and eat four to six smaller meals instead. The larger your meals are, the higher your blood sugar levels rise, which causes your body to release a larger amount of insulin, the "fat storage" hormone, into your bloodstream. That insulin surge overrides any desire by your body to burn fat and instead signals it to store more of the calories you've eaten as fat. Dividing up your meals into smaller portions (such as having a smaller breakfast, lunch and dinner, with small snacks in between) keeps your blood sugar levels even throughout the day so your body releases less insulin, thereby burning instead of storing fat.

DON'T . . . CUT out breakfast. Kicking breakfast to the curb—or eating something small instead because you're too busy—is the biggest mistake men make. That's because missing that first meal of the day not only leaves you feeling hungrier as the day goes on, but it causes most men to eat the bulk of their daily calories at night. The problem? Research has shown that most overweight men consume 60–75 percent of their daily calories in the evening, when their metabolism has already begun to slow down. This makes your body more susceptible to storing all those extra calories as unwanted body fat.

Eating enough calories early in the day—starting with breakfast—not only gives you more time throughout the day to burn them off, but it gives you enough all-day energy to do so. Plus, your metabolism is more revved up in the morning, making it more likely that you'll burn off a lot of those early morning calories before they have time to settle anyplace else on your body.

DO . . . CUT down the size of your plates. A lot of guys don't think about portion sizes when they sit down for a meal; they simply think in terms of filling up their plate. By putting away larger plates and substituting them with smaller ones, you'll end up eating less than usual, even if you finish off everything on the plate.

DON'T . . . CUT out fiber. Research has shown that men that added just twelve grams of fiber to their diet each day dropped one-quarter off their waistline without changing anything else in their diet. That's because foods that are naturally high in fiber tend to have fewer calories, and they take up more space inside your stomach, leaving you feeling full after every meal, so you end up eating less. For the best results, try adding between twenty-five to thirty-five grams of fiber to your diet each day—from fresh fruits and veggies, beans, oat bran, whole grain pasta, brown rice, oatmeal, etc.

DO . . . CUT out the white stuff. A study performed at Tufts University found that men who ate white bread on a regular basis were heavier than those men that didn't. That's because calories from refined grains—such as white bread—tend to find themselves along the waistline (unlike the calories that come from many other types of foods). Instead of eating white bread, switch to whole grain breads instead—you'll not only lose weight, but they're also packed with substantially more vitamins and minerals, plus they contain more fiber, which can fill you up faster and leave you eating less.

DON'T . . . CUT back on water. In fact, I urge you to drink sixteen ounces of water at least ten minutes before every meal or snack. Many men think they're hungry, but many times it's really their body's way of telling them it's thirst. That's because being thirsty activates the exact same physical reaction as hunger. Having some water before you eat may just get rid of your craving, or at the very least leave less room in your stomach for food.

Keeping yourself well hydrated also helps your digestive system do its job more efficiently. By drinking plenty of water with each meal—and all day long—you'll make your digestive system better able to absorb a greater percentage of nutrients from food and move it faster through your body, so you absorb fewer calories that could turn into unwanted fat. Drink at least ten to twelve eight-ounce glasses of water each day.

DO . . . add up each leg that was *CUT* off. The next time you're thinking of eating any common form of meat found in your average supermarket (chicken, beef, fish, etc.), there's an easy way to remember which has the least amount of cholesterol and fat. The more *legs* an animal once had when it was alive, the more fat and cholesterol you'll be adding to your meal. Cattle and pigs both have four legs each—and also the most amount of fat. Chicken—or any type of poultry, such as duck, turkey, etc.—all have two legs (wings not included) and offer even less fat and cholesterol. That's why fish (with no legs to speak of) are the lowest in both fat and cholesterol. (The only exceptions to this rule would be the more uncommon forms of game meats, such as bison, venison, buffalo, etc. Each has far less fat and cholesterol than beef and pork and can be as lean as chicken and fish, depending on the cut.)

did you know that . . .
Your body burns between .8 to 1.2 calories just digesting one gram of protein (which is only 4 calories to start with). That means that by the time you've eaten the protein, about 25 percent of those calories are already used up. A single gram of carbohydrates is also 4 calories, but the reason they are more easily converted to body fat is that your body only burns .2 to .4 calories digesting one gram, leaving 3.6 to 3.8 calories (per gram) lying around after you eat.

"I'm no longer bored with working out."

WILLIAM TAYLOR   AGE: 45 York, PA

"Whenever I'd start to exercise, I'd get bored easily doing the same thing over and over and over again. I tried using a treadmill. I tried riding an exercise bike, but nothing kept my attention. When I hit 45, I finally decided to do something about my shape for health reasons and tried the Body Cuts program. The routine gave me enough variety so I never lost interest. In fact, I actually found myself enjoying exercise for the first time. I'm 19 pounds lighter—and counting—my clothes are beginning to fit a little looser, I have more stamina and my outlook on life has never been better."

did you know that . . .

It takes twelve to fifteen minutes from the time you start eating for your stomach to send a signal to your brain? To give your brain time to turn off your hunger, try to slow things down by either drinking a sip of water after each forkful, talking to friends between bites or simply eating for a minute then getting up to do a quick task before returning to your meal. You're more likely to feel full much faster and end up eating less than usual.

DON'T . . . CUT the wrong corners when it comes to cooking. Picking the right way to prepare your meal can shave off excess calories and fat without changing the ingredients of the meal. Instead, use the following gauge to decide the smartest, healthiest way to cook your foods. Then, think about every meal you eat, see where it ranks and see if it's possible to prepare it using a method that ranks higher on the scale, which is ranked from best to worst:

Steamed
Smoked
Broiled
Baked
Stir-fried
Sautéed
Fried
Deep-fried

Cut Your Risk of Cancer

PICKING THE RIGHT healthy foods to eat won't reduce just your waistline, but also your risk of many of the cancers that afflict older men. Here are my top picks for keeping your body lean and, more importantly, cancer-free:

Broccoli

It's not only one of the most nutrient-dense foods you can eat—teeming with vitamins and minerals—it's filled with isothiocyanates, compounds known to reduce your risk of lung and esophageal cancer by preventing the damaging effects of carcinogens and accelerating how quickly your body can get rid of them. Research has also shown that men who have two or more servings of broccoli a week lower their risk of bladder cancer by 44 percent compared to those who eat less than a single serving weekly.

Tomatoes

Whether you slice them or dice them, fresh tomatoes contain ample amounts of lycopene, a proven antioxidant that's been shown to lower the risk of heart disease and certain other diseases and cancers. They're also filled with other cancer-protecting vitamins, including vitamins A, C and E—all enemies of cancer-friendly free radicals.

Spinach

Extraordinarily high in vitamins A, C, B_6 and E, riboflavin, folate, magnesium, potassium, thiamin and lutein, spinach has been shown to be a valuable tool against liver, lung, colon and prostate cancer.

Garlic

Known to help prevent both stomach and prostate cancer, that little bulb contains a compound known as allyl sulfur that helps slow down and possibly prevents the spread of cancerous tumor cells.

Soybeans

Abundant in muscle-building protein, these tasty legumes also contain isoflavones, a phytoestrogen that may lower your risk of prostate cancer.

Apples

No matter which kind you pick, this fiber-rich fruit helps lower cholesterol and contains flavonoids, the enzymes that attack free radicals that damage your DNA and cause many different forms of cellular damage. It's also been shown that apples contain quercetin, a phytochemical that may be even better than vitamin C at gobbling up free radicals to combat cancer.

Carrots

Loaded with fiber, plus beta-carotene and vitamin A—two natural boosters that improve your immune system and your vision—new research has revealed that carrots also contain falcarinol, a natural pesticide proven to reduce cancer in rats by one-third and which may have the same benefit in men.

Hot red peppers

The same compound that makes you sweat eating them (capsaicin) has also been shown to cause apoptosis—a process where cancerous cells self-destruct by shrinking in size, then breaking up into smaller pieces that the body can dispose of naturally.

Green tea

Not only is each cup rich in powerful cancer-fighting antioxidants, studies have linked this wonder drink to preventing heart attacks, lowering your levels of bad cholesterol, preventing blood clots, easing arthritis and even destroying the bacteria that cause tooth decay.

"CUT" OUT YOUR STRESS

SHOW ME A MAN WHO HASN'T DEALT WITH SOME SORT OF STRESS IN HIS LIFE AND I'LL SHOW YOU A MAN WHO HAS NEVER LIVED

It doesn't matter whether you're young and working your way up the corporate ladder or retired after reaching the last rung and looking forward to your golden years. It doesn't matter if you're a newly crowned father or a grand-dad who gets to sit back to watch his grown-up kids making the same mistakes he did in his youth. Every action and every sacrifice that you've ever had to make for yourself, your family, your career and your life—and every decision you continue to make—each comes with a little (or in some cases, a lot!) of stress attached to it. It's the downside that comes with striving for a better life.

It's also what could be affecting your health right now.

Stress—and its effect on your body—may very well be the biggest threat you face each and every day. Research has shown that stress may be a contributor to the increased risk of heart disease and strokes in men and women alike. That's because subjects dealing with long-term stress tend to have elevated blood cholesterol, elevated blood pressure and blood platelets that tend to clot more often. Countless studies have shown that even small amounts of stress—if not managed—can be unhealthy to your body, leading to everything from minor health conditions like constant headaches and digestive problems, to more major issues like diabetes and unnecessary weight gain.

That's right. Having elevated levels of cortisol—the hormone your brain releases to combat stress—in your system from chronic stress has also been shown to make men fatter. Studies have shown that high levels of cortisol can slow down your metabolism, make you crave unhealthier fatty, salty and sugary foods, plus trigger a response that makes your body store more body fat around your middle.

"I always feel comfortable with Cuts."

JAMES E. SMITH AGE: 49 Ewing, NJ

"As a diabetic and a stroke survivor, I've had to face many challenges, including regaining control of most of my left side. I needed an exercise program that not only worked to help me regain that control, but one that was also safe enough for me to use, and one that made me feel comfortable and encouraged. The Body Cuts program provided me with exactly that. Working out with guys in my age group, who are just like me, I've already lost over 20 pounds and I'm getting in shape for an upcoming kidney transplant. Not only is it a good, sensible program that helped me reach safe, attainable goals, they provide an environment that makes me finally feel at ease about exercise."

Thankfully, there are four major things you can do to ease your stress, reduce your cortisol levels and get your health back to normal. If you're following the Body Cuts program—and the chapter on nutrition—you're already implementing two of the most important stress-preventive measures around. That's because experts agree that the four best things you can do to manage stress are start exercising, watch your diet, get plenty of sleep and stretch often.

The first preventive measure—exercise—is one of the most effective stress relievers for your body for many reasons. Besides keeping your blood pressure and cholesterol in check, it release endorphins—a chemical produced in the brain that reduces pain and brings about feelings of euphoria. It also makes you look better, which makes most men less stressed, if some of their anxiety comes from worrying about looking their age.

The second preventive measure—watching what you eat—reduces stress because many of the healthy foods you would turn to for losing weight also help fight the unhealthy symptoms of stress. Fruits, vegetables, whole grain foods, lean meats, etc., all contain an abundance of micro- and macronutrients—including antioxidants—that help reduce and reverse the dangerous effects of stress on your body.

That leaves two other important players that can prevent stress from hurting your health and robbing you of the results you'll see from the Body Cuts program. But don't worry—I'm about to show you how to easily add both into your life.

Sleep More and Stress Less

I told you that the Body Cuts program would help you achieve a deeper, sounder sleep. But if you're not getting enough sleep, then taking a closer look at what may be stealing it away is an essential step you should be taking for your health.

Stress is considered by most sleep experts to be the number one cause of short-term sleeping difficulties. But the causes could be a variety of factors, which is why it's always a wise idea to talk to a physician about any sleeping problem that recurs or persists for longer than one week. But here are a few things you should consider:

- It could be your lifestyle. This includes drinking alcohol or beverages containing caffeine in the afternoon or evening, exercising right before bedtime, following an irregular morning and nighttime schedule, and working or doing other mentally intense activities right before or after getting into bed.
- It could be your environment. A room that's too hot or cold, too noisy or too brightly lit can easily be the source of your inability to sleep properly.
- It could be you. A number of physical problems can interfere with your ability to fall or stay asleep. For example, breathing disorders, such as sleep apnea or asthma, can make it harder to get a good night's rest. Arthritis and any other conditions that cause pain or discomfort can also have the same effect on sleep.
- It could be your age. Although older adults are more likely to get sleepy earlier, wake up more often, get less deep sleep and rise sooner because of changes in their biological clocks, the amount of sleep they need never diminishes. However, many sleep problems can occur from any changes in an older person's daily routine and quality of life, from retirement, the death of a spouse, health problems and certain medication.

did you know that . . .
Getting enough sleep also keeps you from snacking on bad-for-you foods? According to research from the University of Chicago Medical Center, men who slept less had a 24 percent increase in their appetite for salty and starchy foods.

So how much sleep is considered enough sleep? Most healthy men need an average of seven to nine hours of quality sleep each day. However, there are some men who can perform on less than that, while others can't function unless they've slept more than that. The best way to know if you're getting enough sleep is to simply look at how you operate throughout the day.

If you have a hard time staying alert during monotonous situations, you probably aren't getting enough good-quality sleep. Other signs can be excessive yawning, being irritable with coworkers, family or friends and/or having a difficult time concentrating or remembering facts.

The secret to better sleep starts with a visit with your doctor, who will first want to ascertain whether there are any underlying problems that are contributing to or causing your sleep problem. In many cases, your doctor will be able to recommend lifestyle changes that can help you sleep, but the following tips may be just what your body needs to get more quality rest starting right now:

- **Avoid caffeine, nicotine and alcohol** in the late afternoon and evening. Caffeine and nicotine can delay your sleep by overstimulating your nervous system. Alcohol, on the other hand, may make you sleepy, but it also prevents REM sleep, making whatever sleep you do manage to get less effective.
- **Establish a regular bedtime routine.** If you're not doing so already, make a conscious effort to go "unconscious" at the same time every day. Try going to bed and waking up at a set time, even on your days off. Being lazy and sleeping in on the weekends or on vacation can sometimes disrupt your sleep cycle for later in the week, making you groggy on the days when you really need your energy and mental alertness.
- **Never use your bed for anything other than for sleeping** and to—yes, I said it—have sex. Lying around in bed to read, watch TV, eat, etc., only makes it harder for many men to relax when they finally turn the lights off and use their bed for sleeping.
- **If you find it hard to fall asleep** after lying in bed for thirty minutes, simply get up and try to do something relaxing (listen to light music, read, just take a few deep breaths, etc.) with either the lights off or on low. You'll find yourself feeling tired a lot sooner than if you'd stayed in bed feeling frustrated.
- **Don't be afraid to nap.** It may seem lazy to some guys, or make you feel old, but research has shown that taking a fifteen- to twenty-minute nap in the early to late afternoon can significantly sharpen your memory, improve

your alertness and help lower your risk of feeling fatigued throughout the rest of the day.

- **Watch when you work out.** For some men, exercising right before bedtime can be a great way to tire them out so they enjoy a deeper sleep. But for some men, it can also elevate their heart rate and make them too energized to relax. If that's you, then try exercising an hour before you usually feel that afternoon lull in your day. You'll be more alert and active during the day from the boost, which may help you sleep better at night.

Stretch More and Stress Less

The final, most important preventive measure against stress is simply keeping your body loose and relaxed with some regular stretching. When you're under stress, many muscles—especially the ones located throughout your neck, lower back, and shoulders—tighten up, which can lead to headaches and other unnecessary aches and pains. All of which can be reduced—or eliminated—by stretching on a daily basis.

But stretching goes beyond just relieving stress. Many men simply have no idea how much of a difference stretching can make in every aspect of their lives, especially men in their forties, fifties, sixties and beyond. Regular stretching is designed to alleviate many of the problems men face once they hit middle age, from stiff backs and sore muscles to poor circulation and lack of energy.

It can even recorrect the alignment of your spine by loosening up the tight muscles that tend to pull your back out of alignment. By stretching, you can actually improve your body's posture, which can help you stand straighter, look taller and breathe deeper, giving you extra energy throughout the day. Plus, because it's also a form of exercise, stretching helps lower your blood pressure as well.

As a source of newfound energy and increased flexibility, it's easy to see how stretching can bring new life into old pastimes, whether it's staying quick on the tennis courts, keeping your back limber on the links, playing with your kids and/or grandkids or simply

did you know that . . .
Just taking a few deep breaths every few hours is one of the fastest and most effective ways to lower stress hormones—including adrenaline and cortisol—and feelings of depression? Try sitting upright and taking five to six deep breaths in through your nose and exhaling through your mouth. To get more from every lungful, place your hand on your belly so you can feel it rise and fall—if it's not, you're probably breathing through your chest and cheating yourself of energy-rich oxygen and all its stress-busting effects.

The expression "no pain, no gain" isn't the way to gauge your workout's effectiveness? You need to pay attention to your pain. Experiencing muscle soreness during or following a workout is normal—in fact, it means you're getting a good workout. That's because contracting a muscle past its threshold causes waste material and other acids to build up inside of it. However, if you feel a muscle begin to cramp, stop what you're doing and gently stretch the muscle until it unwinds itself. If you feel any sharp, continuous pain during exercise or pain that persists after a few days, stop the program and get yourself a proper checkup by your doctor to be on the safe side.

recharging an aging libido. The only hard part is knowing the best stretches to use. That's where we've got you covered.

The Cuts Fitness For Men head-to-toe stretching plan is ideal for working out all the kinks the average man deals with throughout the day. The entire plan focuses on and loosens up every major muscle group, including many of the areas that most men never spend time keeping limber and regret later—such as the spine, hips and groin. Best of all, the entire routine only takes five minutes total from start to finish—and that's including the seconds you'll spend in between each stretch changing your body's position to prepare for the next one. Combined with the Body Cuts workout, it's the perfect two-part plan to keep you feeling—and functioning—like a man half your age.

To do the plan, run through each stretch once (as described), then move onto the next stretch in the exact order given. If you would like, repeat the entire cycle of stretches either once or twice, depending on how much time you have.

How often should you use the plan? The good news is as often as you like. Unlike regular strength training and cardiovascular exercise—which require you to take rest days in between sessions—you can stretch every day if you have the time. In fact, the benefits of stretching only multiply if you devote more time to doing it. Try using the program several times throughout the day—such as first thing in the morning, as a midafternoon pick-me-up and right before you head to bed.

However, if you barely have enough time in your day as it is, you should know that sticking to a three-times-a-week schedule is more than most men ever do. Either stretch on the same days that you use the Body Cuts workout—preferably afterward, when your muscles are already warm and more pliable from exercise, or stretch on your off days in between.

> If you're not using the plan immediately after using the Body Cuts workout, warm up your muscles first with 1–3 minutes of a low-intensity cardiovascular exercise, either by jumping in place or briskly walking around your room.

THE CUTS FITNESS FOR MEN
HEAD-TO-TOE
STRETCHING PLAN

Stretch	Move
1	Neck Stretch
2	Shoulder Stretch
3	Chest Stretch
4	Upper Back Stretch
5	Arm Stretch
6	Lower Back Stretch
7	Abdominal Stretch
8	Spine Stretch
9	Hip Stretch
10	Groin Stretch
11	Hamstring Stretch
12	Quadriceps Stretch
13	Calf Stretch

NECK STRETCH

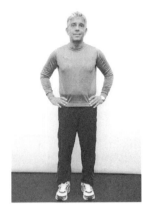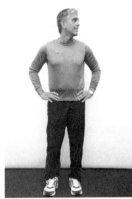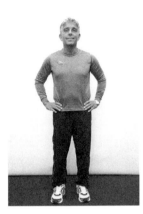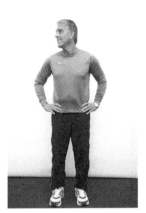

1. Stand up straight with your hands on your hips and your head facing forward.
2. Keeping your body facing forward, gently turn your head to the left as far as comfortably possible. Hold the stretch for 1–2 seconds.
3. Bring your head back to center, then repeat the stretch by turning your head to the right as far as comfortably possible. Hold the stretch for 1–2 seconds.
4. Bring your head back to center, then finish the stretch by tilting your head back as far as you comfortably can. Hold the stretch for 1–2 seconds.

SHOULDER STRETCH

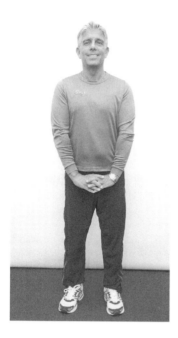 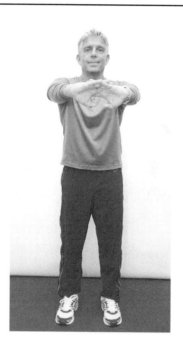 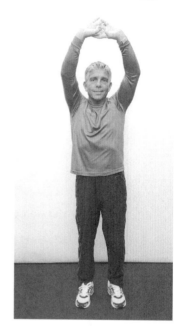

1. Stand straight with your feet shoulder width apart.
2. Clasp your hands together by interweaving your fingers, then twist your hands so that your palms face forward.
3. Extend your arms in front of you until they're straight and hold for 5–6 seconds.
4. Keeping your arms straight and hands clasped together, gently draw your arms up over your head and pull them back behind your head as far as comfortably possible. Hold for another 5–6 seconds.

CHEST STRETCH

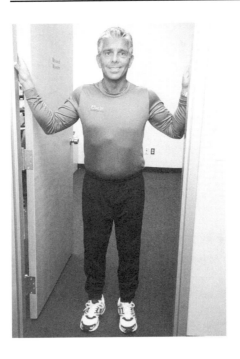 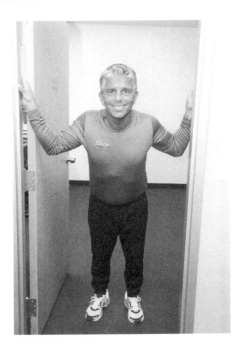

1. Stand inside a doorway and place your wrists on either side of the doorway (about shoulder height).
2. Keeping your feet in place, slowly lean forward until you begin to feel a comfortable stretch along the sides of your chest. Hold this position for 3–4 seconds.

UPPER BACK STRETCH

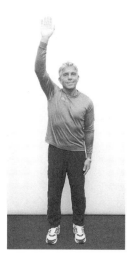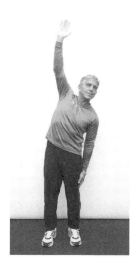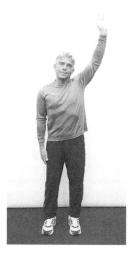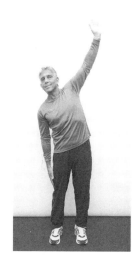

1. Stand with your back straight, knees unlocked and feet wider than shoulder width apart.
2. Rest your left hand flat along the outside of your left thigh and extend your right arm straight over your head, palm facing forward.
3. Slowly lean your body to the left, letting your left hand slide down toward your ankle as far as you can. Hold this pose for 4–5 seconds.
4. Bring yourself back up, switch arms, this time resting your right hand on your right leg and extending your left, and repeat the stretch, this time leaning to the right. Hold for 4–5 seconds.

ARM STRETCH

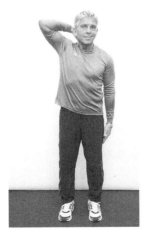 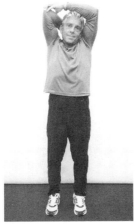 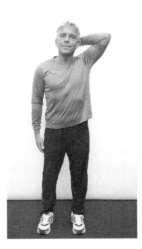 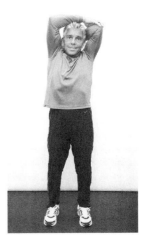

1. Stand up straight and raise your right arm vertically above your head.
2. Bend your right arm so that your right hand drops down behind your neck—your right elbow should be pointing up toward the ceiling.
3. Grab the back of your right elbow with your left hand, then gently pull it back and toward your left shoulder. Hold the stretch for 2–3 seconds.
4. Switch arms and repeat the stretch on your left arm. Hold the stretch for 2–3 seconds.

LOWER BACK STRETCH

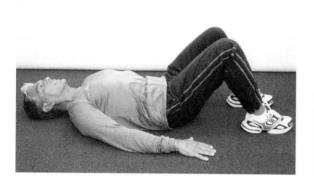 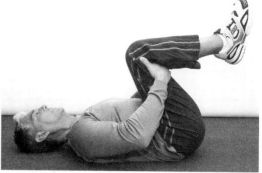

1. Lie flat on your back on a bed—or a soft mat—with your legs bent and your feet flat on the floor.

2. Draw your knees up to your chest, then gently grab just behind your knees with both hands.

3. Exhale as you slowly pull both knees into your chest as far as you comfortably can, keeping your back flat on the bed as you go. Hold the stretch for 4–5 seconds.

ABDOMINAL STRETCH

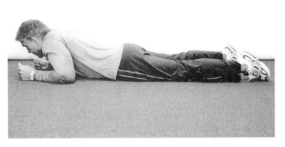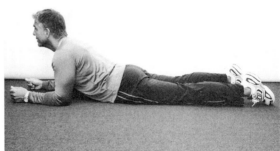

1. Lie on the floor, flat on your stomach with your arms bent—your hands should be up by your shoulders, your forearms flat on the floor and your elbows facing back toward your feet.
2. Keeping your fists on the floor, gently curl your upper body up off the floor—your hips and legs should stay put.
3. Once you feel a gentle stretch across your stomach, hold this pose for 5–6 seconds.

SPINE STRETCH

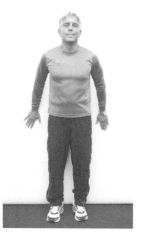
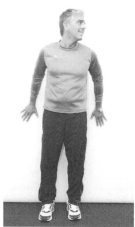
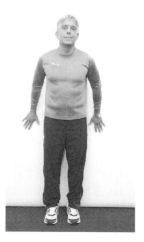
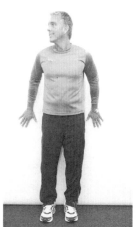

1. Stand with your back to a wall and your heels about six inches away from it.
2. Keeping your feet flat on the floor, gently twist your body to the left as far as you comfortably can and place your hands flat on the wall.
3. Holding this pose, gently push your hips in toward the wall. Hold the stretch for 5–6 seconds.
4. Repeat the stretch, this time twisting to the right instead. Hold for 5–6 seconds.

HIP STRETCH

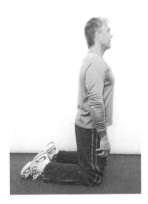 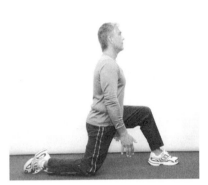 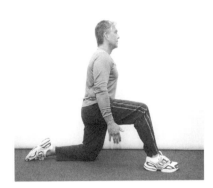

1. Get in a kneeling position with your back straight and arms at your sides.
2. Leaving your left knee on the floor, take a large step forward with your right foot and plant it on the floor in front of you. (Your right leg should now be bent at a 90-degree angle; your knee directly above your foot.)
3. Gently lean forward into your right leg, placing your hands on the floor for support, then push your hips down until you feel a stretch in your hips. Hold for 4–5 seconds.
4. Repeat the stretch a second time by stepping forward with your left foot— your right knee will stay on the floor. Hold for 4–5 seconds.

GROIN STRETCH

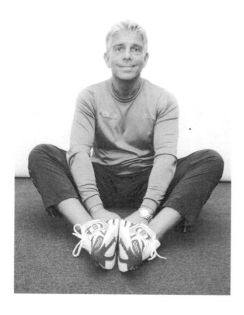 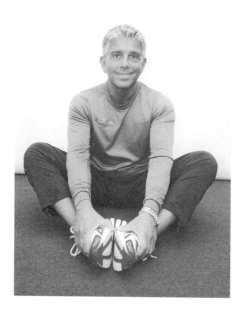

1. Sit down on the floor, bend your legs and touch the soles of your feet together—your knees should end up pointing out to the sides.
2. Reach with both hands, grab your feet and gently pull them in toward your groin as far as you comfortably can.
3. Holding this position, place your elbows on top of your legs and gently press down.
4. Hold this stretch for 8–10 seconds.

HAMSTRING STRETCH

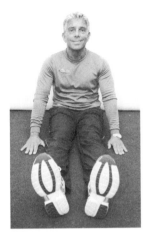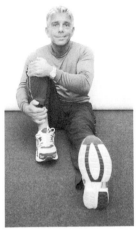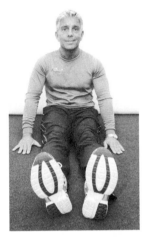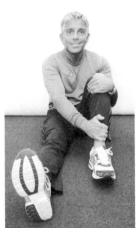

1. Sit on the floor with your legs extended straight out in front of you.
2. Bend your right leg in toward you and grab the outside of your right ankle with your left hand.
3. Gently lift your right foot and slowly bring it toward your body. As you go, grab the outside of your right knee with your right hand.
4. Gently pull your lower right leg toward your chest until you feel a comfortable stretch in the back of your right leg. Hold the stretch for 5–6 seconds.
5. Slowly lower your leg back down and repeat the stretch with your left leg. Hold the stretch for 5–6 seconds.

QUADRICEPS STRETCH

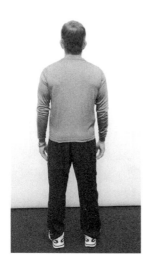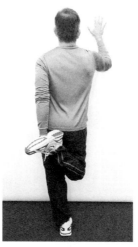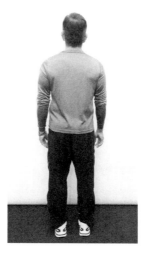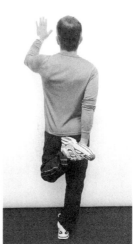

1. Stand a few inches away from a sturdy wall and place your right hand on it for support.

2. Bend your right leg so that your right foot rises up behind you toward your buttocks. Reach back with your left hand and gently grab it.

3. Keeping your right knee pointing down at the floor, slowly pull your right heel in toward your buttocks as far as you comfortably can. Hold for 3–5 seconds.

4. Gently release your foot back down to the floor and repeat the stretch with your left leg. (This time, raise your left foot and grab it with your right hand.) Hold for 3–5 seconds.

13 CALF STRETCH

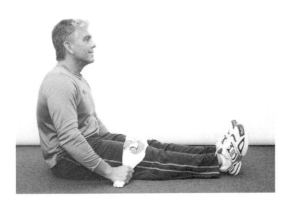 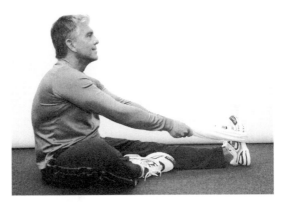

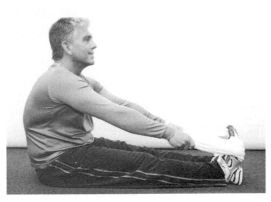 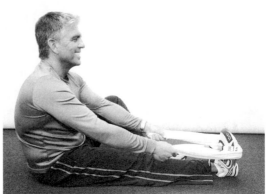

1. Sit on the floor with your legs straight in front of you.
2. Bend your right leg and place the sole of your right foot on the inside of your left thigh—your left leg should end up flat on the floor.
3. Grab a long towel at both ends and loop it around the ball of your left foot.
4. Keeping your back and left leg straight, gently pull back on the towel and bring your toes toward your knees. Hold for 5–6 seconds.
5. Release the stretch, then switch positions to work the right leg. Hold for 5-6 seconds.

Stretching:
The Only Rules You Need to Know

BEFORE YOU START to pull and push yourself around, you have to know the basics first. Here are a few suggestions on how to get the most from the Cuts Fitness For Men head-to-toe stretching plan:

- Take your shoes and socks off. This will give you more stability for holding a stretch, plus being barefoot naturally allows you to relax more.
- Wear nonconstrictive clothing. T-shirts, shorts or sweats are all perfect attire that allows you to stretch comfortably without any binding.
- Use a mirror whenever possible. Being able to see yourself will allow you to check your form and make sure you're stretching properly.
- Take your time. Some of the stretches may feel awkward at first, but just stick with them. Flexibility takes patience, but it eventually pays off down the road. If a stretch hurts, you may be trying to go beyond your limits. Just listen to what your muscles are telling you and you'll never push yourself harder than you should.
- If you need to, feel free to modify the stretches a bit by holding them for less time.
- Breathe as deeply and slowly as possible through the nose. Each breath should come from the belly and not from the chest. The more air you take in, the more oxygen you bring into the body. But go slow. The slower you breathe, the faster you'll relax your body and mind.

"CUT" OUT SOME TIME FOR YOUR HEALTH

IT'S NO SECRET THAT MEN AND DOCTORS GENERALLY DON'T MIX

Why we're so stubborn about seeing a doctor can come from a variety of factors. It's not our fault that we tend to be more embarrassed if the problem is related to something personal, such as depression, sexual issues or anything related to certain areas of our bodies (such as the colon, prostate, etc.). It's not our fault that we tend to grin and bear any aches and pains we may have because of how we've been brought up, believing that having an injury or ailment is a sign of weakness or age. It's not our fault that we're not used to seeing a doctor regularly throughout our lives—unlike women, who make seeing a doctor a habit throughout their teens, twenties and thirties because they have to see a gynecologist.

Or isn't it our fault?

According to research, the fact of the matter is that men visit doctors half as often as women do each year. According to other studies, men also tend to experience heart attacks ten years before women do, are twice as likely to die from skin cancer and we generally live seven to ten years less than the fairer sex. The point is, if you don't think there's a direct connection between not seeing a doctor and not being in better health, you're fooling no one but yourself.

"The Body Cuts program helped me beat diabetes."

TERRY ADAMS   AGE: 61 Hanover, PA

"Before I started using Cuts Fitness and the Body Cuts program, I was 281 pounds. When I went to my doctor for my regular checkup, he told me that my blood pressure was high and my blood sugar was so far out of line that I'd have to start taking insulin right away. When I asked him to give me six months to change things on my own through a better diet and exercise, he reluctantly agreed. That's when I found Cuts Fitness. Six months later, I lost 30 pounds, my blood sugar is back on track and my blood pressure is normal. I am so grateful for finding Cuts when I did and know I'll be using the program forever."

The Body Cuts program will make that trip a lot easier by keeping you in your best shape possible, lowering your odds of hearing any news that you may be afraid to hear. However, sometimes the best way to get over your fear is understanding it from top to bottom. A routine trip to the doctor doesn't have to be painful, especially not if you know what to expect.

Here's a breakdown of what you can expect to hear from your doctor—and what you should tell him so that you hear nothing but great news the next time you see him:

Before the exam . . .

Be ready to tell your doctor everything you know about your own medical history—including details about your diet, your exercise regime, how much you drink or smoke, your family's health history and any symptoms you may be having recently or have had in the past. The more information you can give him, the more angles your doctor can look at when it comes to your overall health and what's best for you.

During the exam . . .

You'll be given a simple examination, which includes taking your height, weight and blood pressure, plus inspecting your ears, mouth, lymph nodes (in your throat) and skin for any unusual markings. Your doctor will also listen to your pulse, lungs and carotid artery (to check for heart murmurs or any blockage in your lungs). Some physicians may also inspect your thyroid and rectum and touch your abdomen for any abnormalities. All of these are painless procedures.

After the exam . . .

Your physician should be honest with you about any health risks you may have and what options you have. Those options might include a change in your current lifestyle, plus whichever lab tests he may feel you need to check on certain health concerns. Those tests could run from checking for heart, liver, kidney and blood problems, to assessing your risk of having diabetes, sexually transmitted diseases, tuberculosis and prostate cancer.

How to Get More from Every Exam

The number one reason most men hate going to the doctor is simple: they hate having lack of control. It's that fear of the unknown that keeps a lot of us from going to see a physician as often as we should, but it doesn't have to be that way.

The good news is that making sure you make the most out of each exam can be a tremendous help. Knowing beforehand what types of tests you *should* be asking for—and at what age—can give you a stronger sense of control the next time you have to see a doctor. The sooner you see one, the sooner he can do his job at spotting and stopping any health problems you may be at risk of before they ever start. Here's my "in control" checklist that every man should follow:

did you know that . . .
Reaching for a toothbrush after every meal could help you lose weight? Researchers in Japan found that men who brushed their teeth after every meal were more likely to be leaner than men who brushed less often. Why? It could be that having fresh breath makes you less inclined to ruin that feeling with more food.

If you're 20 to 29 . . .

- Once a year: Get a blood pressure test.
- Every 3 years: Get a full physical exam.
- Every 5 years: Get a tuberculosis test.

If you're 30 to 39 . . .

- Once a year: Get a blood pressure test, a digital rectal exam (DRE) and a PSA (prostate-specific antigen) blood test—both check for prostate cancer.

- Every 1–2 years: Get a full physical exam.
- Every 5 years: Get a tuberculosis test.

If you're 40 to 49 . . .

- Once a year: Get a blood pressure test, a digital rectal exam (DRE) and a PSA (prostate-specific antigen) blood test.
- Every 2 years: Get a full physical exam.
- Every 3 years: Get an electrocardiogram—especially if you have a family history of heart disease or high cholesterol.
- Every 5 years: Get a sigmoidoscopy—an examination of the rectum—to detect colorectal cancer.

If you're 50 years or older . . .

- Once a year: Get a full physical exam, as well as a blood pressure test, a digital rectal exam (DRE) and a PSA (prostate-specific antigen) blood test. Also, ask for a hemoccult (a test that looks for blood in your stool, which can detect possible colorectal cancer).
- Every 3 to 4 years: Get an electrocardiogram, plus a sigmoidoscopy.
- Every 5 years: Get a full colonoscopy, especially if you have a family history of colon cancer.

Cut Your Odds

THE BENEFITS OF regular exercise extend a lot further than most men ever expect. Here are just a handful of health risks that using the Body Cuts program will help you minimize in the long run:

Arthritis
The Body Cuts program strengthens all of the muscles that surround and support your joints, which can have a major impact on reducing swelling and pain. It also improves your overall circulation, helping your body send vital nutrients to the cartilage along the ends of your bones.

Colon cancer
Regular exercise has been shown to lower your body's level of prostaglandins—the substances found in the cells along your bowels that may be linked to colon cancer. In men that had colon cancer and beat it, exercise was also shown to decrease thier odds of any reoccurrence by up to 50 percent.

Depression
Research performed at the University of Texas in Austin found that even a single session of exercise—roughly thirty minutes' worth—could make a huge difference in reducing depression in the short term. In fact, according to Duke University, exercising three times a week for thirty minutes was found to be equally effective as taking depression medication when performed for at least sixteen weeks.

Diabetes
Dropping just 10 percent of your body weight—if you're overweight for your height—can make a huge impact on reducing your risk of becoming diabetic, since 80–90 percent of all diabetics are considered overweight. Working out also helps the insulin in your body lower your blood sugar levels more efficiently. The two benefits combined can create a tremendous defense against diabetes. The 2001 Diabetes Prevention Program study by the National Institutes of Health revealed that men who performed some form of moderate exercise on a weekly basis lowered their risk of developing type-2 diabetes as much as 58 percent.

Gallstones

Although genetics and yo-yo dieting play a more important role in whether or not you may be at risk for developing gallstones, research has shown that vigorous exercise (the exact prescription of the Body Cuts program) can reduce a man's risk up to 25–28 percent.

Heart disease

Using the Body Cuts program regularly increases your circulation, enlarges your arteries and creates new blood vessels throughout your body. All three benefits contribute to boosting the amount of oxygen that your heart receives, plus help to break down and prevent blood clots from forming. That's why a study performed at the Harvard School of Public Health found that men who strength trained at least thirty minutes a week lowered their risk of coronary heart disease by up to 23 percent.

High blood pressure

Exercising between sixty and ninety minutes a week (the exact length of the Body Cuts program) has been shown to lower high blood pressure by an average of twelve points (systolic) and eight points (diastolic). In fact, a recent study performed in Italy measured the effects of six weeks of exercise, performed three times a week, on patients with high blood pressure. Afterward, their average systolic blood pressure dropped from 143.1 to 135.5 mmHg while their diastolic pressure went from 91.1 to 84.8 mmHg.

Osteoporosis

Women may be four times more likely to develop this condition, but over 2 million men suffer from osteoporosis as well. The Body Cuts program helps to increase your bone density through strength training, which can decrease your risk of spine, hip and other bone-related fractures.

Prostate problems

It may not treat prostate cancer, but researchers at UCLA's Jonsson Cancer Center found that regular exercise—along with eating a low-fat, high-fiber diet—has been shown to slow down the cell growth of prostate cancer by as much as 30 percent. Other studies have shown that men who are active for two to three hours weekly have a 25 percent lower risk of developing benign prostatic hyperplasia (an enlarged prostate) compared to inactive men.

"CUT" OUT SOME TIME FOR YOUR TICKER

The Cuts program may be ideal for improving your cardio-vascular health and burning calories and unwanted body fat. However, adding a few extra activities to your weekly schedule can help you reach your immediate goals that much faster.

Turn Your Free Time into Fitness

Walking, running, cycling and swimming are just a few ways to add cardiovascular exercise into your day, but they aren't your only choices. And you don't always need any high-tech stationary equipment at your disposal to raise your heart rate and burn off a few calories. The good news is that any activity that elevates your pulse and works multiple muscle groups qualifies as cardiovascular exercise.

Here are just a few unassuming ways to keep your heart healthier and the weight off:

- **Be a kid again.** Playing with your kids, nephews, nieces or grandkids lets you do many calorie-burning activities that you would never dare try in public by yourself. Many popular playground activities, from hopscotch to swinging back and forth on a swing set, offer tremendous aerobic benefits. If you think about how quickly kids can tire you out, it's easy to see how trying to keep up with them might be the fastest way toward improving your health.

- **Clean up after yourself**—and everyone else. There's a reason why a lot of guys don't like to pick up after themselves—it's actually hard work. In fact, vacuuming alone burns roughly 230 calories an hour (the same amount you burn walking at a normal pace of 3 mph). Spending an hour doing normal household chores (dusting, taking out the trash, mopping, etc.) won't just score you points with those of the female persuasion, it'll also burn a sizable number of calories off (between two hundred and three hundred per hour, depending on the mix of activities) at the same time.

- **Never take the easy route.** Whether it's the escalator, elevator, the automated walkways in the airport, the drive-by window at your bank, etc.—try to avoid anything that makes things easier on your body or prevents you from keeping your body in motion.

- **Move around when you're standing still.** A study performed at the Mayo Clinic found that sedentary individuals put on eight times more weight (when asked to eat an extra one thousand calories daily) than subjects who also ate extra calories but tended to fidget throughout the day. Whenever possible, try to stand up and pace, even if it's only a couple feet back and forth—you can do it on the phone, watching sports, etc.

- **Park the car as far away as possible.** Instead of spending a few minutes driving in circles looking for a parking space that's right next to where you're going (work, the store, etc.), park as far as possible from the store so you're left with no choice but to burn calories getting there and back.

- **Make a few extra trips.** The next time you load up your car shopping for food, home repair materials, etc., don't load up your arms with as many bags as possible so you only have to make one trip from the car to your house. Instead, grab one bag in each hand and make as many trips as necessary. It's not only better for your back, but it could help you break an unexpected sweat.

Finding the Right Zone for You

As you already know, I prefer that you keep your pulse between 60 and 70 percent of your MHR when performing the Body Cuts program. It's a range that most experts—and all of my clients—find to be the most effective for burning fat and improving your health. However, depending on your goals, there are different benefits that can come from maintaining a lower—or higher—heart rate while using the program.

If you're looking for more of a challenge—or a reason to slow things down a bit—here are all four heart rate zones and the effects that each can have on your health:

HEALTHY HEART ZONE
(50–60 PERCENT OF YOUR MHR)

If you would rather go slow using the Body Cuts program, that's still fine. Maintaining your pulse at 50–60 percent of your MHR is an ideal level for motivating sedentary people to exercise. This low-intensity zone raises your pulse just slightly over your body's natural resting heart rate (the pace at which your heart pumps when you're not active.) This may sound easy, but this basic range is considered physical activity that can still prevent many of the same illnesses and provide many of the same health benefits that exercising at 60–70 percent can —if you stay dedicated to it for at least three times a week.

"Cuts Fitness changed my life."

Cuts SUCCESS STORY 1,494

RICARDO PEREZ AGE: 50 Glendora, CA

"Since using the Body Cuts program for men, I've lost 23 pounds and lowered my body fat 3.5 percent so far. Simply put, this plan has changed my life."

FAT BURNING ZONE (60–70 PERCENT OF YOUR MHR)

This is the recommended target heart rate to use with the Body Cuts program. Keeping your pulse at a steady 60–70 percent of your MHR asks more from your muscles, which is why it's the perfect zone for burning fat. Maintaining this pace also forces your body to use a higher percentage of stored body fat as fuel, instead of relying on mostly glycogen—your body's private stash of stored carbohydrates—as energy instead.

AEROBIC ZONE (70–80 PERCENT OF YOUR MHR)

Revving your pulse up to 70–80 percent of your MHR not only burns more calories, but it challenges your heart and lungs even more, making both of them healthier and stronger. Hitting this zone on a regular basis can also help you see even more health benefits, especially when it comes to reducing your risk for any cardiovascular-related diseases. However, it's a pace that many older men sometimes find hard to maintain, so try it only after using the Body Cuts program comfortably for four to six weeks.

RED LINE ZONE (80–90 PERCENT OF YOUR MHR)

Maintaining your pulse at 80–90 percent of your MHR may seem like a great idea for even further results, but this high level of intensity can be too stressful on the body for many average exercisers—regardless of age—and can actually increase your risk of developing an injury. It's a zone that can hurt you more than help you, which is why watching your pulse is so important as you exercise. If you ever find yourself in this zone when using the Body Cuts program, slow down or stop immediately, wait for your pulse to drop to around 60–70 percent of your MHR, and jump back into the program—but using a less intense pace.

Find Out What Zone You're In— Instantly

LOOKING TO CHANGE the pace of the Body Cuts program, but don't feel like doing the math to make sure you're in the right zone for your goals? This easy-to-use chart can help you quickly figure out if your workout is right on track with your goals. [Caution: I've listed the "Red Line Zone" numbers just to make it easier for you to recognize when you may be pushing yourself too hard. DO NOT, under any circumstances, maintain an intensity or pace that leaves your pulse (beats per minute, or bpm) reaching anywhere within this zone or higher!]

AGE	MHR	HEALTHY HEART ZONE (50–60%)	FAT BURNING ZONE (60–70%)	AEROBIC ZONE (70–80%)	RED LINE ZONE (80–90%)
25	195	97 up to 117 bpm	117 up to 136	136 up to 156	156 up to 175
30	190	95 up to 114 bpm	114 up to 133	133 up to 152	152 up to 171
35	185	92 up to 111 bpm	111 up to 129	129 up to 148	148 up to 166
40	180	90 up to 108 bpm	108 up to 126	126 up to 144	144 up to 162
45	175	87 up to 105 bpm	105 up to 122	122 up to 140	140 up to 157
50	170	85 up to 102 bpm	102 up to 119	119 up to 136	136 up to 153
55	165	82 up to 99 bpm	99 up to 115	115 up to 132	132 up to 148
60	160	80 up to 96 bpm	96 up to 112	112 up to 128	128 up to 144
65	155	77 up to 93 bpm	93 up to 108	108 up to 124	124 up to 139
70	150	75 up to 90 bpm	90 up to 105	105 up to 120	120 up to 135
75	145	72 up to 87 bpm	87 up to 101	101 up to 116	116 up to 130
80	140	70 up to 84 bpm	84 up to 98	98 up to 112	112 up to 126

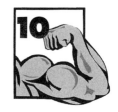

CUTS FOR LIFE

ALMOST EVERYONE WANTS TO BE IN BETTER SHAPE, SO WHY AREN'T MORE MEN DOING SOMETHING ABOUT IT?

Sometimes, it's not about having enough time to sweat it out or having access to the right types of equipment. There are still plenty of other things out there waiting to put an end to your exercise before it begins. Staying motivated throughout the entire week—especially on the days when exercise may be the farthest thing from your mind—and preparing your days wisely so you can stop excuses from creeping into your workouts are two important concerns to help keep you from falling off the workout wagon before you even get going.

Plan Right . . . and Exercise Forever

As you continue to use the Body Cuts program, the results alone that you—and others around you—will begin to see happening to your body should be enough to keep you inspired to exercise. But dodging obstacles before they start is easy, if you remember these simple motivational tricks:

"Finally, a plan that builds better muscle— and not just bulk."

KARL SCHLICHTING AGE: 73 Covina, CA

"To be honest, the main reason I work out is vanity. But the problem I've always had with other workout plans is that they're designed for guys looking to get bulky. The Body Cuts program lets me get a full-body workout in less time, but what I like is how it lets me be more physically and mentally fit."

- **Plan your workout** as if it was an important meeting: write it into your daily schedule, then work the rest of your schedule around it. Treating exercise like important business will teach you to treat it with the importance that it deserves.
- **Always be ready to exercise.** Instead of letting forgetfulness mess up your workout plans, keep a full set of exercise clothes—shirt, shorts, shoes and a towel—in both your car and where you work. That way, you'll always be prepared to sweat. Or stick your workout clothes in front of the things that cause you to skip workouts—like on top of your TV or overtop your favorite snack, for example. You'll be less likely to skip a day when you're forced to move your workout clothes to get to your guilty pleasure.
- **Exercise on the busiest day of the week.** If you can plan to work out on the worst day of your week, you'll find you have fewer excuses when you need enough motivation to carry you through a hundred easier days.
- **Do it for someone else.** The next time you feel inclined to miss a workout for a particular excuse—too much work, feeling tired, etc.—remember that the healthier you are, the more able you'll be to be there for the ones you love. As soon as you think of bailing on exercise, immediately picture those that depend on you.
- **Prioritize your life.** Track your time for a week—down to the very hour— writing down every single thing you do. After the week's over, grab a few different colored highlighters and spend a few minutes highlighting each hour according to what you were doing at that moment. Use blue for goofing off, red for work, yellow for family time, orange for any physical activity, green for sleep, etc. When you see how much blue time you really have in your life, it's easier to see how you may be wasting the time you could—and should— be using for other important things, such as exercise, enough sleep, etc.

- **Bet a friend that you won't quit.** Money doesn't just talk; it's also perhaps the greatest motivator when it comes to sticking with exercise. There's a classic study that asked a group of subjects to bet $40 that they could stick to a long-term exercise regime of three thirty-minute aerobic workouts a week for six months. Of the subjects who risked their money, 97 percent were successful in sticking with the program, while those subjects who didn't risk their money were only 20 percent successful.
- **Give yourself a performance bonus.** Many guys are more motivated to work harder at their jobs when they know there is a possible bonus waiting for them if they reach a certain quota or goal. Try doing the same thing with exercise. Think of something that you really want but are hesitant to buy (a rich meal, a new golf club, etc.) and attach some sort of attainable goal to that item (dropping a pant size, losing five pounds, etc.). Knowing there's something you *really* want attached to a healthy goal that your body *really* needs can make it easier to focus on the prize and not on how hard it is to get the work done.
- **Make a deal with your wife and kids.** This works in a similar way to the "performance bonus" tip I just shared with you, only instead of trading goals for gifts, try exchanging workouts for chores. Make a deal with your family each and every week that you'll stick with the Body Cuts program and exercise three times a week. If by the end of the week, you've stuck to the program, then someone else has to do one of your chores instead of you—maybe it's doing the dishes or taking out the trash for a week. If you miss a day in the week, then you have to do one of their chores instead (make it a chore you *really* hate and you'll be more likely to never miss a workout).

"It's so easy to look and feel better in less time."

Cuts
SUCCESS STORY
1,823

DAVID GLAVAN AGE: 24

"Finally, I've found a quick, yet effective workout style that I feel I can recommend to anyone trying to get their lives together and get in shape while maintaining a busy schedule. So far, the results keep coming and my body fat has dropped nearly 5 percent so far. I have much more energy, feel much better than ever before and can honestly say that I enjoy using the Body Cuts program. Who else can say that about exercise?"

The Next Cuts Success Story: You!

Throughout this book, I've been able to share with you just a few of the success stories I've received from countless men whose lives have been transformed using Cuts Fitness For Men and the Body Cuts program. I've even been able to share my own. But there's still one success story that's missing:

Yours.

You now have all the tools that I—as well as thousands and thousands of men just like yourself worldwide—have used to feel and look younger, put on lean muscle and finally lose the fat. That's why after using the Body Cuts program, the head-to-toe stretching plan and cultivating the rest of the healthy lifestyle habits presented in this book, I want you to track your success and tell us about it.

Please write to me:

Mr. John Gennaro
Cuts Fitness For Men
c/o My Success Story
1120 Raritan Road
Clark, NJ 07066

Just as with many of the testimonials in the book, telling us your story doesn't have to be much word-wise. Even a few sentences can be extremely inspirational—especially when read by someone who shares the same issues or problems that you do. Sometimes I share similar success stories with members or people I meet who I think would be interested in hearing that they're not alone with their fitness goals and their personal dilemmas.

Who knows? Just as I've hopefully inspired you to turn back the clock using the Body Cuts program, the very next guy to be inspired to change his life for the better through exercise may do so entirely because of you.

Stay healthy and enjoy every minute of your new life.

Keep Track to Stay on Target

No matter which Body Cuts workout you use—in the gym, at home or on the road—the best part about all three is that you never have to worry about writing down how many repetitions you perform of each exercise. All you need to do is run through all sixteen exercises a total of three times. That may make it a lot easier to monitor your workouts, but that doesn't mean you shouldn't track your progress on a regular basis.

Making sure that you perform all sixteen exercises three times in every workout is essential to the program. Making sure you exercise three times a week is just as crucial. To monitor both areas, these two checklists can help. As you perform each exercise or workout, just mark it off on the chart with an "X" and you'll always know if you're following the Body Cuts program to the letter.

WEEKLY WORKOUT CHECKLIST

DAY ONE

	Exercise	Set #1	Set #2	Set #3
#1				
#2				
#3				
#4				
#5				
#6				
#7				
#8				
#9				
#10				
#11				
#12				
#13				
#14				
#15				
#16				

WEEKLY WORKOUT CHECKLIST

DAY TWO

	Exercise	Set #1	Set #2	Set #3
#1				
#2				
#3				
#4				
#5				
#6				
#7				
#8				
#9				
#10				
#11				
#12				
#13				
#14				
#15				
#16				

Cuts FITNESS FOR MEN

WEEKLY WORKOUT CHECKLIST

DAY THREE

	Exercise	Set #1	Set #2	Set #3
#1				
#2				
#3				
#4				
#5				
#6				
#7				
#8				
#9				
#10				
#11				
#12				
#13				
#14				
#15				
#16				

MONTHLY SCHEDULE

	MON.	TUES.	WED.	THURS.	FRI.	SAT.	SUN.	TOTAL
Week #1								
Week #2								
Week #3								
Week #4								
Week #5								

A FINAL NOTE

Since you've made it this far, you probably already know that the Cuts Fitness For Men program was created to change lives. In the four years since I first developed this program, I've had the privilege of watching thousands of men of all ages, sizes and backgrounds transform their bodies and their lives using the Cuts system. Until they discovered our program, many of these men felt left out of the world of fitness and exercise. They wanted to look and feel better and more alive, but they didn't have a way in, a place to begin. Now they feel in charge, in shape and more in control—it's a great feeling, and one I want to share with as many people as possible.

Leading a healthy lifestyle is actually quite simple once you have the understanding, motivation and basic tools. Through our franchise locations, and with this book, I hope I've helped you take action toward living a longer, healthier and happier life. Taking 30 minutes, three times a week to exercise and lead a healthy lifestyle should now be a priority for you. I hope you'll embrace this system—and in the process, truly thrive, inside and out.

In good health,

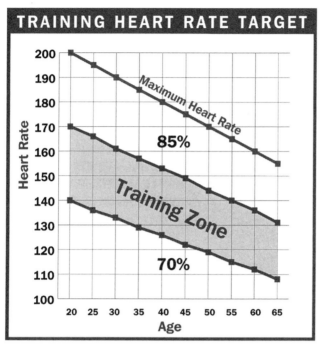

TRAINING HEART RATE TARGET

Maximum Heart Rate

85%

Training Zone

70%

Heart Rate

Age

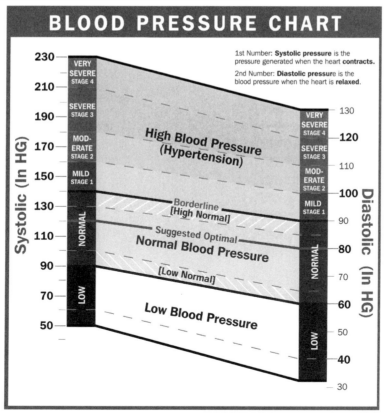

BLOOD PRESSURE CHART

1st Number: **Systolic pressure** is the pressure generated when the heart **contracts**.

2nd Number: **Diastolic pressure** is the blood pressure when the heart is **relaxed**.

Systolic (In HG)

VERY SEVERE STAGE 4
SEVERE STAGE 3
MOD-ERATE STAGE 2
MILD STAGE 1
NORMAL
LOW

High Blood Pressure (Hypertension)

Borderline [High Normal]

Suggested Optimal
Normal Blood Pressure

[Low Normal]

Low Blood Pressure

VERY SEVERE STAGE 4
SEVERE STAGE 3
MOD-ERATE STAGE 2
MILD STAGE 1
NORMAL
LOW

Diastolic (In HG)

ADDITIONAL RESOURCES

American Diabetes Association: www.diabetes.org/risk-test.jsp?WTLPromo
=corporate_risktest
Take the risk assessment to find out if you are in danger of getting diabetes.

American Heart Association: www.americanheart.org
Take the "Learn & Live" quiz to find out about your risk of getting heart disease.

CNN Health Library for Men: www.cnn.com/HEALTH/library/men
Take a look at the Diagnostic Tests section for great explanations regarding common health tests.

Cuts Fitness For Men: www.cutsfitness.com
Check out the latest Cuts Fitness For Men news, locate a franchise or view our products.

Food and Drug Administration: www.fda.gov
Get information on the latest FDA news, recalls and safety warnings.

Kids' Health: www.kidshealth.org
Great overall health resource for both kids and their parents.

Mayo Clinic: www.mayoclinic.com/health/mens-health/MC99999
Visit the Men's Health Center for quick health diagnosis information.

MSN's Fitness Section: www.msnbc.msn.com/id/3034511/
Check out the comprehensive daily articles and advice on a variety of fitness topics.

***New York Times* Health Section:** http://nytimes.com/pages/health/index.html
Enjoy terrific writing on important health news in an easy to read format.

Real Age: www.realage.com
Take the Real Age Test and find out the biological age of your body.

ACKNOWLEDGMENTS

First and foremost, I need to give thanks to Gary Heavin, the founder of Curves, for creating a wildly successful women's fitness franchise over the last fifteen years that provided me with the inspiration to create something similar for men in my hometown of Clark, New Jersey.

To our Cuts franchisees, I will never be able to express the great respect and gratitude I have for all of you in helping us truly blaze the trail for men's fitness. It has not been easy, but I am sure that you all will agree that it has been a fulfilling experience knowing that you've provided a product that has changed many lives for the better. I hope that you are all extremely proud of this book, as the foundation was written based upon your experiences and the successful results and passion of your members.

I also owe special thanks to the extraordinary contributions of Steven Haase, my business partner and my friend, who has been instrumental in the formation and growth of our company, as well as the components of this book. Steven, we have a lot to be proud of, and special thanks to your family—Nadine, Kayla and Alec—for all of their support as well. Thanks to Bryan Healy, our director of fitness and training, who helped me create the first Cuts Fitness For Men franchise in an old camera shop in Clark. Bryan, it's been quite a ride, huh?

Special thanks to Myatt Murphy, one of the premier fitness writers around, who brought this book to life. At Perigee, I had the pleasure of working with Marian Lizzi, our editor, who had the foresight to contact us after having great success with the

Curves book. Marian, your insight and intelligence have made this a better book. Thank you. And last, but certainly not least, I need to thank my family—my brothers Joe and Gary, who have both provided me with lots of love and support over the years. We have come a long way from Newark, huh?

To my mom and dad, who are both angels in heaven, you are always in my heart and always on my mind. I hope that you are as proud of this book as I am. To Louisa, my baby dog, thanks for your unconditional love and support. To anyone I have missed, I'll mention you in our next book. Thank you all.

INDEX

Page numbers in *italic* indicate figures; those in **bold** indicate tables.

busiest day of week, exercising on, 142
Buxton, Brent, 100

Cable Curl, **36**, 49, *49*
caffeine and sleep, 110
calendar, tracking workouts, 31, **147–50**
Calf Stretch, **113**, 126, *126*
cancer, foods for reducing risk, 105–6
capsaicin, 106
carbohydrates, calories used in digesting, 103
cardiovascular exercise, **16**, 16–17, 28
carrots, cancer risk reduction, 106
cereal for lunch or dinner, 137
Chair Dip, **79**, 84, *84*
Chair Squats, **79**, 87, *87*
checklists
    exercise, 146, **147–50**
    "in control," doctor exams, 131–32
Chest Press, **36**, 37, *37*
Chest Stretch, **113**, 116, *116*
cholesterol, 13–14, 17, 108
chores, exchanging workouts for, 143
clothes for exercise, 96, 142
colon cancer, 133
colonoscopy, 132
commonsense eating, 101–4
compound exercises, mix of, 30, 31–32
cooking methods, 104
cortisol, 108, 111
Curl Press, **56**, 70, *70*
Curves, 4
Cuts Fitness For Men, 3–23
    cardiovascular (aerobic) exercise, **16**, 16–17, 28
    contact information, 144
    doctor exams, 129–34
    doctor visits as needed (goal), 11, 22–23, 29
    excuses for not exercising, 5, 53
    goals every man should have, 10–23, 28–29
    growth of, 4, 6
    Head-to-Toe Stretching Plan, 111–27, **113**
    heart health, 135–39, 151
    Home Workout, 31, 53–73, **56**
    injury risk reduction, 13, 34, 35
    motivation, 96, 141–50
    muscle vs. fat, 12–13, 17, 29
    necessity of, 6–8
    No-Excuses Workout, 31, 75–96, **79**
    nutrition, 99–106, 108
    Official Body Cuts Program, 31, 33–52, **36**
    resources for, 154
    sleep eight hours a night (goal), 11, 21–22, 28–29

strength (resistance) training (goal), 11, 12–14, 28, 30, 76, 101
stress reduction, 107–11
waist-hip ratio (goal), 11, 19–20, 29
website for, 54
    See also Body Cuts Program; maximum heart rate (MHR); pulse

day off between workouts, 30–31, 32
deal (making) with family, 143
depression, 133
diabetes, 133
diastolic blood pressure, 134, *153*
diets, failure of, 100–101
digestion, calories used in, 103
digital rectal exam (DRE), 131, 132
doctor exams, 129–34
doctor visits as needed (goal), 11, 22–23, 29
"dodging the doc," 22
dopamine, 55
Double Crunch, **56**, 71, *71*
DRE (digital rectal exam), 131, 132
Dumbbell Fly, **56**, 59, *59*
Dumbbell Lunge, **56**, 60, *60*
Dumbbell Press, **56**, 57, *57*
Dumbbell Row, **56**, 72, *72*
Dumbbell Squats, **56**, 64, *64*
Dumbbell Triceps Extension, **56**, 61, *61*

easy route, avoiding, 136
eating, 99–106, 108
electrocardiogram, 132
endorphins from exercise, 108
energy cycle of body and exercising, 73
energy from stored fat and calories, 100–101
equipment for
    home workout, 54
    no-excuses workout, 76, 77
exams, doctor, 129–34
excuses for not exercising, 5, 53
exercise adherence, 6
extracurricular activities caution, 73

falcarinol, 106
falling asleep problems, 110
fat burning zone (heart rate), 16, **16**, 138, **139**
fat storage hormone (insulin), 102
fiber, importance, 102–3
flavonoids, 106
flexibility, 34, 111–27, **113**
foods, "Cut" out the bad, 99–106, 108
Foster, Melvin, 20

ABOUT THE AUTHORS

John Gennaro is the president and founder of Cuts Fitness For Men. Gennaro brings an extensive background of more than twenty-five years in the health and fitness industry and is the former creator of the internationally successful Abs on Air, as well as many other fitness products—selling more than five million units via cable infomercials. He founded Cuts Fitness For Men in May of 2003.

Myatt Murphy is the author/coauthor of five popular exercise and nutrition books and a frequent journalist for more than forty-five magazines worldwide, including *Esquire*, *Fitness*, *GQ*, *Men's Health* and *Self*. For more information on his books, go to www.myattmurphy.com.

Steven Haase is the managing director of Cuts Fitness For Men. His background includes a unique blend of marketing, education and strategy. He was also the founder of Princeton Learning Systems, the pioneer of online education.

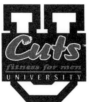

KEEP ON LEARNING,
AND GETTING IN SHAPE,
WITH CUTS FITNESS UNIVERSITY

WE'VE ALL HEARD that fitness is good for us, but few of us truly get the most out of our fitness regimens, because our knowledge of how exercise really works only goes skin-deep. Throughout this book, I've tried to give you a solid working knowledge not just of what to do to get in shape, but also what your body needs to thrive, and why.

In keeping with the Cuts mission to educate as well as offer a great workout experience, I've started something called Cuts Fitness University. Under the direction of our managing director, Steven Haase, who was the real pioneer of corporate online learning in the mid-1990s, the university will offer essential, easy-to-understand information about health and fitness that you can use to lead a healthier life *now*. Minicourses are designed by the Cuts Fitness team as well as leading organizations such as the American Council on Exercise.

Sample topics include the following:

Strength Training 101
Commonsense Eating
Knowing Your Maximum Heart Rate
Ready To Run?!
Visiting Your Doc

I invite you to take a look at the Cuts University website at www.cutsfitness.com/university. I hope you'll agree that it offers the type of lessons that will keep you on the road to good fitness and great health.

Sincerely,

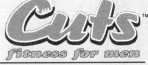